Opioid Reckoning

OPIOID RECKONING

Love, Loss, and Redemption in the Rehab State

Amy C. Sullivan

University of Minnesota Press
Minneapolis
London

The publication of this book was assisted by a bequest from Josiah H. Chase to honor his parents, Ellen Rankin Chase and Josiah Hook Chase, Minnesota territorial pioneers.

William Brewer, "Overdose Psalm," from I Know Your Kind copyright 2017 by William Brewer. Reprinted with the permission of The Permissions Company, LLC on behalf of Milkweed Editions, www.milkweed.org.

More information is available on the book's accompanying website, https://mnopioidproject.com.

Published by the University of Minnesota Press
111 Third Avenue South, Suite 290
Minneapolis, MN 55401–2520
http://www.upress.umn.edu

ISBN 978-1-5179-0863-8 (hc/j)

Library of Congress record available at https://lccn.loc.gov/2021025889

Printed in the United States of America on acid-free paper

The University of Minnesota is an equal-opportunity educator and employer.

28 27 26 25 24 23 22 21   10 9 8 7 6 5 4 3 2 1

For my girls, with love

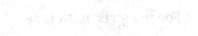

Overdose Psalm

For how long and why I cannot say,
But in the wake of the great spruce falling,
everything—the axe, its weight in my chapped hands,
the skirt of golden trunk shavings,
the tree like an overturned ship—
is so altered by light, so foreign,
I can't believe it's what I was after,
if I was after anything. And to think
I would survive? It can't be, though,
as is so often the case, it is: the column
of light breaking through the black woods
only a reminder of what once resisted it.
I'm beginning to think that resistance
is everything, how it kept what is now
trees leading to a clearing, a forest.
Snow committing its slow occupancy,
filling the column like words, the light
saying in so few of them, like all terrible
truths, something here did not survive.

—William Brewer

Contents

Prologue

One cloudy October Sunday in 2011, I came downstairs later than usual, happy to have slept in. I stopped at my daughter Madeleine's room to close her door before I started coffee in the adjacent kitchen. As I reached for the doorknob, I glanced in and noticed she was in a peculiar position: sleeping like an infant with her butt in the air, she was facing my direction with one cheek half scrunched on her laptop keyboard. Closing the door, I noticed that she looked a little peaked. My night owl must have been up late.

Moments later, over the coffee grinder's whir, I heard her yelling for me. I ran to her room. "What? What is it, honey?" She was crying, and her eyes were completely panicked and her lips dry and wrinkled. With clenched fists and limbs pulled taut into her stiff little frame, she looked blue-grey-pink, like the colors of a just-hatched baby bird.

"What's going on, sweetie, where do you hurt?"

"I can't move! Momma! I can't move my leg. I can't *feel* my leg! Momma! Help me!"

I looked more closely around her bed. A huge, wet stain covered her sheet where her mouth had just been—and a needle with an orange syringe a few inches away. A needle. Frantic, angry, and scared, I held the needle near her face, "What did you do? What was in this?!" Contrary to the evidence, she replied, "It's not mine."

I ran to the stairs and called frantically for my husband. I heard him bound from bed, and he was down with us in seconds, dressed and ready to go. He went into her room, lifted her up into his arms, and we headed to the car. Coiled up in the back seat, she cried, moaned, and asked repeatedly for water, but she could barely hold it without spilling all over herself. She looked worse with every passing minute. I wondered if we should have called an ambulance, but it all happened so fast, and we were halfway there already. We went to the hospital we knew, not the one that was closer—adrenaline and shock are powerful forces.

When we arrived at the hospital emergency room, I jumped out of the car for help. A female attendant took one look at her and rushed back inside for a gurney. Within a few minutes, we were answering questions and digging for insurance cards. We did not know what she took or what had happened the night before. I had put the needle from her bedroom in a baggie and brought it along, but no one cared or needed it here: the evidence was her body. The ER doctor was able to get her wavering and weak attention, but she was still disoriented and seemed to have trouble hearing. He very loudly asked her what she took.

"Heroin." Her voice was scratchy and coarse.

I was both furious and frightened. Heroin? I stayed in the room, watched nurses start IVs, insert a catheter, and hold bags to her face as she vomited. She smelled acrid, musty, bitter. They cut her T-shirt off. Cut off her sweatpants and dropped it all in the trash. She couldn't stop crying about the pain in her leg. As they rushed her down the hallway for an X-ray, I took a picture of the bag of urine hanging off her bed—it was the color of black tea, the color of kidneys failing, as I would learn later. Somehow in that moment I needed evidence for what I was experiencing, for the disaster happening right now to my daughter.

I went to the waiting room. Soon a nurse came and handed me a clear plastic bag with Madeleine's necklace in it, a simple piece of red thread with an infinity charm attached. My sister had given one to each of us the Christmas before. We all made wishes as we tied one on each other's wrist or neck. What was her wish then, I wondered, as I took the bag from the nurse.

A few minutes later I decided to walk down to see if she was back from the X-ray. The curtains were closed in the now crowded room—I could see many feet moving around. People were shouting information and orders, and then the sound of an electric thump made my knees buckle. Instead of falling, I leaned back into the cold, tile wall and slid slowly to the floor. The nurse who had brought me the necklace peeked behind the curtain. Someone else came with a chair for me. *Oh, god, she's dying.* Another hollow, powerful thump followed. More commands. In the hall, someone said gently to me, "Her heart stopped, but they've revived her. Her heart's beating again." I glanced in, only to see a ventilator tube, more IVs, cords and bags, and another catheter, this one in her neck. For the next twelve days, my dear daughter would be silent. A machine would do her breathing for her, but I didn't know that yet.

Our youngest daughter, Lucia, not quite fourteen, was at a school retreat that week about a hundred miles away. I knew she would want to come back, and when I called, a teacher offered to drive her to the hospital right away. I waited for her outside now, grateful that she did not experience what I just had.

After her cardiac arrest, the medical situation had apparently escalated beyond the scope of that hospital on that particular Sunday, so the ER doctor and administrators made the decision to transfer her to the county hospital's Level I trauma unit. Thankfully, Lucia arrived soon after this decision was made, because within minutes, an EMT team had Madeleine in an ambulance headed to what was then Hennepin County Medical Center (now Hennepin Health). We followed in our car.

By the time we arrived, several people were already focused on my daughter's situation. HCMC is a renowned teaching hospital—I only remembered this after seeing so many scrubs and white coats in the room. A resident pulled back the sheet to reveal that her right leg had swollen to twice the size of her left one. The chief medical doctor, a sweet professorial type—even wearing a sweater vest, for god's sake—asked me in astonishment, "Why didn't they say anything about her leg?"

"I don't know. It didn't look like that a couple hours ago. I hadn't seen her leg. They took X-rays and a CT scan. . . ."

He asked me to describe how I found her. He nodded. "She's got acute compartment syndrome." Two health assistants were taking her jewelry off, removing nose rings, piercings, gingerly putting the little balls and metal pieces in biohazard bags. He explained patiently, "The right leg had no circulation for several hours due to her being too passed out to move naturally as we do when our blood flow gets cut off. When she woke up, the cells in the leg released proteins into her bloodstream and her kidneys could not keep up. That's why she had cardiac arrest and why her kidneys are failing." He said he would check in on her later. I didn't want him to go.

The hospital we had just left was where Madeleine had been born eighteen years ago. This one seemed out of my league—a swarm of activity, instructions, and care. More IVs, cords, monitors, and a respirator were attached to her body in this new place, and soon a group of surgery residents strode in. Lucia and I were still in the room when they started talking about her sister's leg. I should have covered her ears.

"It's been too many hours since this happened; she will likely lose her leg."

"Lose her leg? Why?" I asked.

Very matter-of-factly he said, "It's dying, and much of it is probably dead already." I was horrified. Lucia started crying.

I continued, "So, you are just going to take her leg off, right now, just like that?"

"Well, I am going to talk to the chief surgeon, but yes, probably."

These orthopedic residents were tall, handsome, fit. Their arms were crossed over their chests. They seemed some part intrigued, some part aloof, and from my perspective, not particularly sad about the situation at all. The one who seemed to be in charge said, "I'll be back soon." As he passed me, he quipped that I should be glad she'd at least have her *life*.

I soothed Lucia as best I could. Anxiety combined with waiting so long in one place, powerless to do anything, made my body feel like lead. We found a little conference room and piled in there. When I noticed the same surgery resident sitting at the nurses' station a little while later, I went over to him. "Hi, I would like to talk some more about this. What do you know *for sure* about her leg already being beyond healing? We don't know exactly how many hours she was in that position. Are you sure it has to be amputated?"

He leaned back in the chair, stretched his arms behind his head, looked at me for a second, and then shifted his eyes back to the computer screen. "I'm waiting for the chief orthopedic surgeon to call back. I will let you know what he says." I walked back to the conference room feeling angry, anxious, and powerless in equal measure.

Sometime later—ten minutes or two hours, I don't know—the resident came back with papers for me to sign. "The chief said we have to try to save her leg; she's only eighteen. There may be complications. We are going to open her leg and clean out as much of the dead tissue as possible. If you agree, sign these, and understand that she may not make it through the surgery." Layers of trauma were piling up so quickly.

A nurse kindly escorted us out of the conference room we had commandeered and directed us instead to a beige, polyester-clad waiting room, where we sat numbly, picked at food, and stared up at random nature shows on the grainy television set suspended awkwardly from the ceiling. After midnight, a kind, bespectacled man with a brief-case came into the waiting room. He introduced himself as the chief surgeon and said that her surgery went well, that they had been ag-gressive in removing dead tissue, and that we wouldn't know for some time—forty-eight hours until the next surgery—if the leg was finished dying or free to heal. I showered him with gratitude for trying to save her leg, for not giving up. He said he had to try. "She's only eighteen."

After five numbing, disorienting weeks in what seemed like every wing of the hospital—intensive care unit, cardiac, renal, physical rehabilitation—Madeleine achieved a complete physical and cogni-tive recovery. Within a year, though, her opioid addiction reappeared with a vengeance. Three years later she found the right combination of care for her substance use disorder and has had a healthy, thriving life ever since.

Introduction
Opioids, Oral History, and the Rehab State

Before I ever thought much about stigma, and even less about people who used hard drugs, I was the mother of a struggling teenage daughter. In the year or so before Madeleine's near-death overdose, when she would fall asleep midsentence at dinner, I thought she was overtired. She always stayed up late—maybe she didn't get enough sleep, or maybe she'd smoked some pot. Annoyed, I would suggest she go to bed. I was naive and did not know this "nodding off" was a clear sign of opioid use. I didn't even know the meaning of the word "opioid" then. By her senior year in high school, when she was taking college courses full-time and making straight As, I thought I had done everything I possibly could to help her change course.

Two years earlier, Madeleine had exhibited some extreme-to-us emotional and behavioral issues that made us fear for her safety. Looking back now, I can see this was one of those tipping-point moments; we had her admitted to a hospital-based, dual-diagnosis program for teenagers. After a one-week stay, the psychologist discharging her told us in her presence that Madeleine did not have "an addiction issue" and was mostly struggling with my divorce from her father. Any time after this when I raised my concerns about her pot or alcohol use, she reminded me of his assessment. By the time she was sixteen, we were locked in a power-struggle standoff. Out of a deep fear for her physical safety, I knew that if I forced more treatment or therapy on her, I would lose her—she would flee home and, therefore, safety. I had once imagined those two being intertwined. I did not know until years later the negative impact that one-week hospitalization had on her. She met highly medicated teens struggling with severe mental illness; she learned that the tendency among adults to deploy excessive fear of *all* substance use had the opposite effect on her peers; she figured out that by keeping a calm, low profile at home—not acting out with us—she'd have more freedom and, maybe, could earn more of our trust.

Madeleine's experience in the hospital program, combined with the one damaging family meeting at her discharge, troubled our relationship for years to come. Despite my efforts to be an active and engaged parent, battling the Sturm und Drang (storm and stress) of living with a smart, sensitive, and fiercely independent daughter got harder every year. I had read, studied, and even taught college courses about girlhood, feminist education, and the mounting social pressures on teen girls.[1] I sought out therapists for her and for myself, and I tried to balance freedoms with boundaries, privileges, and consequences. I wanted her teen years to be easier, but hard was what they were. That she used heroin at home in her bedroom shocked me to my core. In fact, I could never have imagined any teenager using heroin, having access to it, or most of all, not being deathly afraid of it.

I grew up in the seventies and eighties, in an era when most teens knew of heroin as an extremely dangerous drug that *killed* people, especially famous musicians and actors. In the mid-1990s, when she was three, I definitely wasn't paying any attention to what was coined "heroin chic" in the fashion world.[2] Even President Bill Clinton weighed in on it, when he remarked that "glorifying heroin" in the fashion industry was "not creative, it's destructive." He was referencing the 1996 heroin-related death of Davide Sorrenti, a prominent young fashion photographer who posed models that looked drugged and gaunt, a new style that had created a buzz in the media.[3] I didn't recall the heroin-related part of the story but vividly remembered the sickly-looking young models with dark makeup under their eyes. I was not impressed; I had those dark circles naturally. Expecting another baby and having just defended my master's thesis in history, I was an educated, middle-class, white mother in a university town in Oklahoma. My world did not yet include girding my children against heroin addiction, or any drug for that matter. Even in the mid-aughts, I was not aware that prescription pill opioid addiction had created a new and much larger market for heroin. When pain pills became both ubiquitously available by prescription and yet more expensive on the street, enterprising drug dealers flooded the new market with cheaper, stronger heroin. They used the I-35 corridor running through the center of the country to distribute heroin in cities and small towns from south to north.[4] My daughter's easy access to opioids had actually been in the works for several years before either of us knew it.

The shock of the years that followed her overdose took a while to coalesce into something tangible and meaningful. The complexity of substance use, addiction, and the multiple methods of treatment for it, when combined with my own white body privilege in an unequal system of racism, stigma, laws, and punishments, challenged me to step out of my comfort zone—to think, talk, and write about some really hard things.[5]

When I discovered William Brewer's collection of poems I *Know Your Kind*, his question in "Overdose Psalm" seemed to be speaking to all of us, my daughter and I, our family, everyone I knew who'd experienced such a scare or such a death. "And to think / I would survive?" She did. We did. We did not lose her. Even after so many years, writing that still makes me take a deep, grateful breath. I see now how her overdose created a "light breaking through the black woods" that Brewer's poem imagines, now "only a reminder of what once resisted it." This book, too, contains the light and the dark, the resistance and the survival, of people who have passed on and of those who still live, strive, and struggle in the context of this oldest of human–plant relationships: human pain and suffering relieved by the ubiquitous, beautiful poppy and all its chemical relatives.

The narratives that comprise this book are based on oral history interviews I conducted over four years that became what I named the Minnesota Opioid Project. The collected interviews were initially born of a personal and scholarly desire to document the lives of mothers I knew and admired through our shared experiences mothering children with substance use issues. After interviewing a dozen of them, as well as a few fathers, I sought out others who were personally affected by the epidemic and/or whose work was connected to it in some way: other family members, addiction-treatment staff and directors, physicians, social-service and public-health professionals, and harm-reduction advocates. The sixty-plus narrators were a diverse group from all walks of life and different parts of Minnesota, from the North Shore of Lake Superior to the Greater Twin Cities metropolitan area; from the White Earth Nation to rural farming communities in western Minnesota.[6] I am deeply honored and humbled to be able to present some of their life stories here. In the face of stigma, ignorance, and despair, their tenacity and bravery continued to resonate with me long after our first meeting.

When I was a graduate history student in the 1990s, the topic I wanted to write about had not yet been written about historically, and the people who were present to it in the 1970s were still alive. I found some of them, and this was how I stumbled upon the practice of oral history.[7] Ever since, oral history has remained the richest source of content for the histories I am drawn to investigate and write about. Oral histories provide deep insights into our understanding of how communities remember and process significant events. They are a gift to the present and the future and help us humanize our collective past.[8] Oral history can also be used to study social problems, document community change, and guide future policy decisions.[9] The aim of this book is to do some of all three. I am particularly driven to dissect and expose stigma against drug users. By preserving the deeply personal histories of people whose lives were affected by opioids, and by interrogating the consequences of the many ways that cultural, social, and medical stigma violates basic human principles of love and kindness, I hope to elevate discussions that often take a victimization view or a criminalization view, depending on the race and class of the users and their families. While I was listening and learning to deconstruct stigma through these narratives, I soon realized I was also capturing stories of trauma, sometimes even seeing how it passed seamlessly through generations.

Oral histories of trauma and addiction are sensitive in so many complex ways, for both the listener and the narrator. They require abundant trust and empathy. As an essential component of an ethical oral history practice, the mutual feelings of trust required in such historically and currently burdened contexts means that projects like this one cannot be rushed to completion.[10] Trust must be earned over time with tenderness and diligence; it cannot be forced or cajoled under deadlines. As a mother with direct, lived experience around the topics my narrators shared, my insider knowledge heightened my ability to earn this trust and to empathize deeply, even when listening to stories about things I could have never imagined experiencing. Tears were shed on many occasions in both directions.

As is the case with oral histories, the more narratives I recorded, the more complex the picture became. The vast, interlocking nature of problems associated with drug use regularly overwhelmed me, but with each interview, I gained a more nuanced understanding of how the opioid epidemic has touched so many aspects of life in the twenty-first century. Some insights presented themselves to me so many times that I saw a painful, almost never-ending pattern emerge: stigma thrives on shame; shame thrives on fear and regret; fear and regret find refuge in silence; silence keeps stigma intact. This cycle is not only an internal emotional one shared by individuals and families, it is also embedded in institutions, laws, and protocols meant to "help" people with substance use disorders.

Although this project focuses on the intimate and individual lived experiences of Minnesotans, it is also important to understand the broader social and market-driven systems that have shaped the contemporary landscape of opioid use. In 2011, the U.S. Centers for Disease Control and Prevention (CDC) declared opioid overdose deaths an epidemic, and the drug in all its forms continues to inflict long-term, widespread damage on families and communities across the nation. Three waves of deaths associated with opioids have been identified, the first beginning in 1999, just three years after the Food and Drug Administration approved prescription opioids in the form of OxyContin, then marketed aggressively by Purdue Pharma. The second wave began in 2010 with a drastic increase in heroin use. The third wave, the one we are still in, began when illicitly manufactured fentanyl hit the streets around 2013.[11] The legal and ethical reckoning with pain pill pharmaceutical giants like Purdue Pharma has only just begun, with states leading the charge against opioid manufacturers.[12] Fentanyl is nearly one hundred times stronger than heroin and pain pills and has been laced into those street drugs and others, killing people in such record numbers that by 2018, illicitly manufactured synthetic opioids accounted for two-thirds of overdose deaths in the United States. Although heroin deaths remained steady in 2019 in Minnesota, synthetic opioid deaths increased by nearly 50 percent, with fentanyl found in nearly all of them.[13]

Opioid-related deaths were so prevalent over a period of several years that life expectancy for *all* Americans decreased as a result; the number of lives lost eclipsed automobile and gun-related deaths. Between 1999 and 2019 more than 500,000 Americans died from drug overdoses involving opioids.[14] Daily media consumers encountered a tragic statistic or story about the epidemic nearly every day. We heard about deaths by overdose in bathrooms, cars, and bedrooms; the emergent "Generation O," young children who lost parents to overdose; legislation efforts to curb access to prescription pills; and the devastating economic and social impact in hard-hit places like West Virginia, Kentucky, Tennessee, and Ohio. These stories appeared in both long-form journalism and sound bites, talk shows, podcasts, and documentaries.[15]

Public health and media education about overdoses even made it to the hallowed venue of Super Bowl commercials for two years in a row and highlighted the new demographic of heroin drug users: young, white, suburban kids.[16] "That's How" depicted the quick bedroom overdose of a male high school athlete, and the following year, "All American Girl" featured the uncertain demise of a dog-walking, blonde, high school cheerleader. These emotionally evocative and sympathetic ads were distributed by the National Council on Alcohol and Drug Addiction (NCADA), but quickly garnered criticism for using fear tactics and for not directly promoting treatment options or harm-reduction interventions. Although the NCADA said it hoped the ads would "ignite conversation about the realities and catastrophic consequences of opioid and heroin use in our community," it is evident watching them that by "our community," they meant affluent, white communities. The ads did nothing to equalize the danger of opioids among racially or economically diverse populations of users.[17]

While public sympathy and media attention focused on children and parents from white, middle- and upper-class homes, the demographics, consequences, and historical realities of opioid users who were not white continued to be criminalized in ways that the War on Drugs had prescribed decades earlier. The rate of opioid use between Black and white Americans is similar, but Black people are six to ten times more likely to be incarcerated for their drug offenses and, in Minnesota, twice as likely to die from an overdose. The authors of one compelling study compared the use of "white opioids"—synthetic opiate pain pills abused by white suburban and rural Americans—to show how drug policy in the United States is highly racialized. As white people began dying in large numbers, science and medicine came to the rescue to decriminalize their addictions, "carving out a less punitive, clinical realm for whites" that made their problem a biomedical one, while "leaving intact more punitive systems that govern the drug use of people of color."[18]

Access to economic and social capital allowed some of the narrators in this oral history project the best kinds of mental health care while others, mostly Black, Latinx, and Indigenous bodies, served jail sentences.[19] Their substance use disorders were the same, but the consequences of addiction remain drenched in racism, moral judgment, and the ignorant-but-comforting notion that "addicts" are just bad people. Another related phrase, "living under a bridge," became an all-too-common way for white-bodied people to distinguish their loved ones from what they imagined stereotypical drug users to be. The fact that drug use is so deeply tied to people who lack housing remains yet another injustice in our country that has become stigmatized as a way to dismiss it. The thinking seems to go that if drug use causes a person to lose access to shelter, and drug use is considered a choice, then it becomes easy to justify the opinion that drug users must *want* to be living on the streets. Wouldn't a lack of shelter also contribute to the escape that drugs provide? Addictions among drug users in urban communities of color or in rural, impoverished white communities are also often assumed to be a consequence of poverty, trauma, and dysfunction. On the other hand, when privileged white bodies use drugs in a dangerous and chaotic way, they are often perceived as becoming addicted by chance, or that one bad choice, or because of drug dealers who preyed upon them. Systemic racism adds another heavy layer to the stigma of addiction and the social discrepancies users face. These entrenched belief systems often grace white people's addictions with medical jargon and pity while criminalizing and incarcerating people of color who use the very same drugs. This is not to say that stigma against drug users and addiction in white communities doesn't exist—it most certainly does—but it will never compare to the damage that communities of color have experienced due to the consequences of addiction in their communities.[20]

What changed during the current epidemic, the reason it got so much more attention and empathy than, say, the crack epidemic of the 1990s, was because white bodies were the ones dying, both rich and poor.[21] These new opioid users were not 1960s-era hippies, outliers, musicians, or artists. Hard-drug users and their parents might still be judged and scorned, but white users had racial and often economic privileges that softened the legal and treatment consequences. In the 2010s, the faces of white suburban kids and, somewhat less so, working-class and unemployed adults in the hollowed-out Rust Belt got the attention and the pity of the press, and ultimately the attention and pity of the country.[22] As Keturah James and Ayana Jordan observe, when addiction affects people of color, it is seen as a "pathological shortcoming," not addressed with treatment but more often with "militarized policing and involvement of the criminal justice system." Even when stories did cover communities of color, racialized stereotypes and stigma remained powerful because, as the authors plainly point out, "this practice of employing a public health strategy for white middle-class groups, but a crime-control agenda in urban minority neighborhoods is deeply entrenched in American political culture."[23] It would come as no surprise then that the attention the epidemic has garnered among vocal, well-resourced families—mostly white—may ultimately contribute to positive, widespread solutions and improved treatment for all people with substance use disorders. No one would argue that this would be a good outcome, but it will only be so if the positive changes are dispersed equitably among *all* people with substance use disorders.

When I began this project, I did not know that a significant portion of the history of alcohol and drug treatment began in the state I now call home. The narrators in this book shared life experiences in their interviews that reflected the distinct histories and deep philosophical differences between the more dominant anonymity- and abstinence-based model (Twelve Steps, "rehab," and AA), the medical model (evidence-based, targeted-population methadone clinics), and street-based, drug user–focused services (harm reduction and syringe exchanges). Given the presence of these three models—and even despite the dominance of AA-based treatment—I wondered if Minnesota could integrate them all and be a leader in the effort to end the trauma and tragedy of the opioid epidemic.

Compared statistically with other states, Minnesota has never been among the most severely affected by the opioid epidemic, but the dramatic increase in deaths was still significant. Between 2000 and 2019, annual opioid-related deaths increased from 54 to 428, nearly 700 percent.[24] The state's overdose death rate has always been among the bottom ten in the nation, yet this number belies the impact on people of color in the state. American Indians comprise just 1.4 percent of the state's population, yet their overdose death rate was seven times higher than among whites. Among African Americans, 6.8 percent of the population, death rates were two times higher than those of whites.[25] Minnesota has one of the most glaring racial disparity statistics in the nation across all social welfare markers: income, education, health.[26] Institutional racism and the criminalization of drug addiction wrecked communities and families for decades before prescription pain pills launched the opioid epidemic. Attributed to poverty, gang violence, and the everlasting War on Drugs, many people of color who were imprisoned or died of overdoses lacked access to proper treatment, and thousands are still serving out excessive sentences, despite an underlying substance use disorder and the related issues that landed them in trouble in the first place.[27]

By 2010, state, local, and tribal leaders in Minnesota began to take the dramatic increase in opioid use seriously. Various constituencies and organizations held town hall educational forums and harm-reduction summits, created an Opioid Dashboard, and passed legislation to increase access to and education about the antidote drug naloxone. The Minnesota Prescription Monitoring Program and later the Opioid Prescribing Work Group created and set guidelines that tracked and encouraged doctors to reduce the number of pain pill prescriptions.[28] The White Earth Nation began hosting an annual Harm Reduction Summit in 2011 in response to the devastating impact injection drug use and overdose deaths were having in their communities.[29] Clinton Alexander, Anishinaabe White Earth Band of Ojibwe, a public health professional with the White Earth Health and Behavioral Health Divisions, was a founding member of the White Earth Harm Reduction Coalition and one of the first organizers of the annual summit. The conference has grown every year since then and gathers tribal health professionals, state and local public health leaders, treatment centers, and grassroots organizers from across the country to share best practices and current information about the impact of drugs, overdoses, and related infectious diseases. In 2019, Alexander Greenfield and Brenna Greenfield, a professor at the University of Minnesota's Medical School–Duluth, collaborated on a nationally funded "HotSpot" fatality review study for an in-depth look at the lives of tribal community members who died from opioid overdoses in order to better understand risks and improve protection and prevention efforts. Both the White Earth and Red Lake Nations' tribal governments have become cutting-edge leaders in the epidemic, employing novel and culturally specific interventions to create systems of care that provide

long-term, wraparound services to increase community health, reduce opioid addiction, and lower the frightening number of overdose
deaths.[30]

The multifaceted approach taken by these various stakeholders
makes sense given Minnesota's history with medical and behavioral
health innovations like the Mayo Clinic and early alcohol treatment
centers like Hazelden. During the late 1940s and early 1950s, the most
prevalent, standardized model for addiction treatment in the United
States emerged in Minnesota among three organizations: Willmar
State Hospital, Pioneer House, and Hazelden, now the Hazelden Betty
Ford Foundation. Together, they coalesced ideas, philosophies, and
methods to create a multifaceted treatment protocol based on several core principles. What we know as residential or outpatient drug
and alcohol treatment was founded in the state and thus came to be
known as the Minnesota Model.[31] Prior to its development, state mental hospitals and inebriate asylums were where the chronically addicted languished, some for the remainder of their lives. Innovations
for psychiatric patient care in the 1940s coincided with a growing dis-
illusionment about traditional treatment for alcoholics as well.[32]

The Minnesota Model was revolutionary because of its approach
and its flexibility, which stood in stark contrast to earlier concepts of
alcoholics as being incurable, or that alcoholism was merely a symp-
tom of other deep, underlying psychological disorders. First among
the model's core ideas was remaining abstinent from alcohol, a goal
maintained by the guiding philosophy of the Twelve Steps of Alcoholics Anonymous. This included attending regular group meetings
as well as fostering a personal spiritual practice that developed or
revived one's relationship with God, often referred to as "a Higher
Power." The model strongly promoted the definition of alcoholism
and drug addiction as a "primary, progressive disease" with "physical, psychological, social and spiritual dimensions."[33] Peer support and
the hiring of recovered alcoholics as counselors was also a novel innovation, as was using a multidisciplinary team for client care that
included clergy, social workers, nurses, physicians, and psychologists
in both group and one-on-one settings. Before leaving treatment, the
goal was to get to Step Four, "Made a searching and fearless moral
inventory of ourselves," or Step Five, "Admitted to God, to ourselves,
and to another human being the exact nature of our wrongs." Post-
treatment, clients were strongly urged to attend regular AA meetings

and continue to "work the Steps," an introspective, self-awareness practice that involves following the moral and spiritual guidance offered in each consecutive step.[34] This treatment model, also known as TSF, Twelve Step facilitation, is world-renowned and the most ubiquitous model in the United States' drug-treatment industry.[35]

Since alcoholism was seen as a chronic condition, abstinence from *all* mind-altering substances was required to maintain sobriety for the rest of one's life. Only while sober was a former alcoholic or "addict" (to use the term of the time) in recovery. "In recovery" intentionally implied that these people were never fully recovered—that was the insidious nature of the disease. If a person relapsed on alcohol or drugs, the start date of sobriety began again at that new day one. For AA-affiliated groups, one's time without using substances, whether it was twenty-four hours or dozens of years, signified success with the program. Going to meetings, following the program, and working the Twelve Steps leads to sobriety and a more fulfilling life. "It works if you work it," the saying goes. Peer support in these self-help, affinity groups is absolutely essential. Historically, the emergence and popularity of these groups marked a profound change in the world of recovery from alcoholism and addiction. The General Services Office of Alcoholics Anonymous estimates that in 2019, there were 71,000 groups and nearly 1.5 million members of AA in the United States and Canada. Since they do not keep membership records, this number is based on reports to the national office from local groups.[36]

The Minnesota Model for drug treatment, in tandem with the ubiquity of Alcoholics Anonymous, has been the origination point for how so many of our common cultural and social ideas of drug treatment are based. A slew of AA slogans and mantras abound, and the repetition of them often reminded me of aspects of my own Catholic upbringing: "Go to meetings. Keep coming back. It works if you work it. Let go and let God. There is no chemical solution to a spiritual problem. Once an addict or alcoholic, always an addict or alcoholic." Even the "disease model" of addiction, while it seems like it would be related to medicine, isn't—the disease concept has long been used as a signifier for the persistent and perpetual nature of addiction's long-term hold on a person, which requires constant vigilance to prevent relapse. Describing alcoholism like an allergy was one of the first steps toward defining addiction as a physiological affliction. Dr. William Silkworth articulated it as an "allergy of the body and an obsession of the mind," believing that those who had this condition should never drink alcohol again. He helped AA founder Bill Wilson understand and then articulate alcoholism as a disease, particularly as one that required confronting the person's ego. The disease concept the Minnesota Model espoused gave chronic substance use a familiar name for what we understand as illness, but also kept the moral aspect of addiction in the mind and soul of the individual.

The Minnesota Model became the standard for the ever-growing drug- and alcohol-treatment industry, with facilities now numbering in the thousands across the country. In the 1990s, the state was even jokingly referred to as "Minnesober" or the "Land of 10,000 Treatment Centers."[37] Getting our child into "rehab" was what I and every other parent I met thought we had to do, no matter their age and no matter how many times they had already been. The common quip was, "It's either treatment, jail, or death." When my daughter was still in the intensive care unit, one of the first terms I heard from someone in long-term recovery was, "I wonder if this is her 'rock bottom.'" This term is ubiquitous among AA and Twelve Step groups. It refers to the point at which an addicted person gets so low and experiences such depths of danger and despair that they finally decide to seek long-term help. I also heard "rock bottom" in the parent support groups I attended. People wondered when it would happen, knowing it was scary, but their voices still resonated with a smidge of hope. We all knew that when the drugs were opioids, "rock bottom" could very likely result in sudden death.

Addiction medicine and research, in particular neuroscience, describes addiction as a chronic but treatable brain disorder. Twentieth-century scientists who researched drug users "discovered" addiction in their labs, most notably at the Addiction Research Center, located on the grounds of the United States Narcotic Farm in Lexington, Kentucky.[38] By the early 1960s, Marie Nyswander and Vincent Dole, two researchers at the Rockefeller Institute for Medical Research, collected routine observational research that showed how a low dose of methadone, an opioid-based pain medicine, when given once a day to heroin users, stopped their cravings and allowed them to resume functional, stable lives. By the late 1960s, methadone maintenance had gained significant ground.[39] Due to a convergence of factors from the 1960s forward, the placement of methadone clinics in cities with high rates of Black heroin users, stigmatized as criminal drug users, meant that methadone as a drug treatment would become associated with "hopeless," urban cases, despite its proven ability to allow people to resume more normal lives.[40] As the opioid crisis grew, two other drugs, buprenorphine and naltrexone, became more widely prescribed by clinics and certain specially licensed physicians, and methadone treatment, despite its stigmatization and extreme federal restrictions, increased as an effective medical treatment for opioid dependence. The physicians I interviewed whose stories appear in this book expand on how the use of medications for opioid dependence had been siloed in the state until very recently—more than a decade into the pain pill and heroin epidemic.

People who use illicit drugs, or use prescription drugs illicitly, have always been among the most marginalized people in our communities. The harm-reduction approach to addiction treatment emerged in the 1980s as a reaction against the prohibition-centered, carceral model that saw all drug users as criminals. It took a more neutral stance about drug use itself, preferring instead to focus on reducing harm and preventing accidental death by overdose. The AIDS/HIV epidemic solidified this philosophy and its person-centered, nonjudgmental approach.[41] Harm reduction as a concept has been stigmatized itself and is perceived by many as permissive and enabling of drug use; I, for one, learned about the opioid overdose antidote naloxone a few years before I knew what harm reduction was.

In 2016, when I began teaching "Uses and Abuses: Drugs, Addiction, and Recovery" at Macalester College, a small, rigorous liberal arts college in St. Paul, I decided to change the perception of harm reduction as "bad" in my classroom by bringing in a local harm-reduction professional, Stephanie Devich, to train my students how to use naloxone. They left class with a naloxone kit. Both Stephanie and I remained committed to the trainings, but I always wondered if any of the kits were ever used. Student EMTs who took my class soon lobbied for campus-wide access and education. Two years later, trainings were offered to the campus community at large by enthusiastic harm-reduction peer educators, the first of whom were trained by Stephanie. The health center agreed to provide kits to students and also placed them in specified emergency locations in the dorms and around campus.

When the COVID-19 pandemic forced us all apart and online, I still wanted to get students naloxone-trained in my classes. During our first online semester, a peer trainer made a video, and I arranged for postal delivery of the kits to my students' now far-flung locations. To my great surprise one night in mid-November 2020, I received an email from a student living on campus who wrote,

> Thought you would be interested to know that I just revived a guy on the bus with the two vials of naloxone you gave me. It was pretty crazy; he was blue and I just drew up the vials and gave it to him! He revived after the second dose and was up and gone before the paramedics arrived. I just wanted to say thanks for handing out the naloxone in your class.[42]

I was stunned by this news. A save! Applied humanities and civic engagement are cornerstones of my teaching philosophy, and yet the thoughtful way that my students so willingly discarded stigma and embraced harm reduction took my teaching and the mission of this book to a whole new level. It matters how we treat each other. It matters how we care for each other.

All of the professionals, family members, and others I interviewed who treat, care for, and love people with substance use disorders are stellar human beings. They, too, want their work to matter in the lives of the people they serve. Because they often embodied different approaches, the history of the push and pull between these models for addiction treatment—abstinence-only versus medical interventions—emerged as one of the key conflicts of this book. How does a state that is the birthplace of "rehab" reckon with highly addictive and very deadly new kinds of opioids? How does the abstinence model continue to justify itself when clients leave treatment and promptly die from an opioid overdose? How can a sober house deny housing to residents who need opioid-agonists to function so they can get their lives back on track? What could harm-reduction practices of the AIDS/HIV era offer to this epidemic of overdose deaths? Why do medications that treat opioid use disorder, like methadone and buprenorphine, remain marginalized, stigmatized, and difficult to obtain, especially during a crisis like this one?

With my own family's experience with opioid addiction lying squarely in front of me, the lives of my narrators guided me through these questions. What emerged were complex answers that highlight their experiences within a historical context. This book is not a history of the current opioid epidemic in the United States nor a history of the War on Drugs. Nor does it present a thorough history of the Minnesota Model, addiction medicine, or the history of research on addiction. Many talented historians and scholars have and continue to chronicle the complexity of this most human affliction. This book is about capturing the stories of people who have interacted and interfaced with the consequences of opioids in a ubiquitous drug-treatment model that has only recently started to embrace medications and harm-reduction services.

The opioid epidemic, the COVID-19 pandemic, and the revived but long-suffering racial injustices we faced in 2020, and most notably for this state, the murder of George Floyd in Minneapolis, have all amplified the deep inequities in our country that have existed for generations now: inadequate access to effective addiction treatment; a profit-driven healthcare system; pervasive stigma; a housing crisis; and the related traumas of racism, violence, and incarceration. The moment is fraught with difficulty and calls for the kind of reckoning this book aspires to. Do not despair, though. There are also plenty of redemptive and empowering stories on these pages. Doing this work has taught me much about our ability to survive traumas of all kinds. The will to live, improve, recover, and innovate is as human as all of our other struggles, failures, and weaknesses.

CHAPTER 1

Mothering Addiction
Lessons in Trauma Parenting

A ll too familiar with treatment centers, emergency rooms, detox facilities, drug court, jails, and maybe even prisons, parents of children with an active substance use disorder live in a parallel but alternate parenting universe. While friends' and colleagues' children graduate from high school and college, maybe get married, and achieve financial independence, these parents navigate rehabs, insurance, sober housing, and the criminal court system. If addiction issues began during adolescence, the normal development of frontal lobe decision-making and discernment abilities may likely be stunted or delayed.[1] Long after most parents have finished the tasks related to raising their children, parents of adult children with substance use disorders will often continue caretaking for many years.

Mothers and fathers become accustomed to living in a state of constant worry and intervention, stepping in to do whatever has to be done *this* time, regardless of the child's age or duration of the addiction. The skills honed as parents—protecting, nurturing, guiding—continue long into adulthood. If extended over many years, the heightened attention to repetitive, impending disasters becomes mentally and physically exhausting, and feels impossible to maintain. All kinds of failures surround them: parenting, treatment, recovery, relapses, deaths. Hope and hopelessness become locked in a constant struggle. The biological, psychological, and social complexity of substance use disorders is overwhelming, and stigma around drug use remains strong, whether spoken or unspoken. One mother, DeeDee Tillitt, who lost her son Max to an overdose in 2016, described the isolation and lack of understanding she felt during her son's active addiction: "I almost wish he would have had cancer because then he would have the best practices and protocols, and people would show up and give us casseroles."[2]

While coping in the midst of the myriad crises connected to addiction, what these parents end up doing might appear to be an aspect of the now common, overbearing "helicopter parenting," but most of their interventions and rescues are based on actually preserving the very lives of their children or, at the very least, trying to keep them from further harm.[3] Parenting a child with a substance use disorder requires a more intense kind of harm reduction that is different from the typical attention to a child's safety and health that most parents practice. They must address a higher level of danger and consequences, life-and-death choices, navigating simultaneous paths of power and powerlessness. This kind of parenting is a deeply complex terrain. The onset of substance use disorder during a child's teenage years sets this pattern in motion, so letting go of these heightened parenting behaviors feels dangerous and irresponsible. But suppose a parent does? Many are advised to do just that by experts and family members alike. What happens to their child then? It is a brutal choice. And with opioid addiction it can be a deadly one.

Over one summer, I interviewed twelve mothers who had a child or children with opioid use disorder. We met in homes and coffee shops; we sat in cars, took walks, and shared meals. The mothers ranged in age from their late forties to late seventies, and they were married, divorced, single, straight, and gay. All of them were white and identified as either Christian, Jewish, or agnostic. Though their incomes and economic backgrounds varied, most had college degrees with careers in sales, nursing, insurance, education, social work, public relations, urban planning, and landscape design. Their children wanted for little in terms of access to attention, resources, and opportunities. In fact, they had a lot in common with other white, college-educated, middle-class mothers whose children never developed ongoing substance use problems.

Although these mothers experienced much of the social and cultural pressures of parenting children with addiction, especially the shame and the blame, they did not give up easily. Their experiences offer testimony about mothering addiction. How did they both witness and weather the trauma and complexity of addiction? How did they navigate barriers to treatment, contradictory professional advice, and the chaos that often follows active addiction? Through the intimacy of long-form oral-history interviews, I hoped to document how they engaged in the all-consuming work of mothering addiction as the opioid crisis worsened by the day. Their tenacity and love never faltered as it chased alongside stigma, miseducation about drugs, and the multiple barriers to effective, evidence-based treatment.

The stories in this chapter represent the experiences of a self-selected group of mothers. The experiences they shared are qualitative, not meant as data but as stories to learn from. When I did add up some of the numbers, though, I learned how even with ample financial resources, white body privilege, and access to treatment, the opioid addictions of their children were not being treated effectively. This group of mothers has thirty-six children among them, sixteen of whom struggled with opioid addiction. Every child's substance use disorder emerged in adolescence. Those sixteen teenage or adult children went to inpatient treatment programs over one hundred times; this number does not include outpatient program attendance, of which there were dozens more. Six or so were in recovery from opioid use, but most of the mothers considered these to be "fragile" recoveries. Between 2007 and 2016, six of the sixteen died from opioid overdoses—two in 2016 alone. Another passed away in 2020. The introduction of fentanyl into the illicit drug market was directly related to three of the overdose deaths among this group.[4]

The opioid epidemic has laid bare the inconsistency of substance use treatment protocols for opioid use disorder, so, sadly, it made sense that the number of attempts at sobriety were so high and that the overdose deaths were, too. Medications available to manage opioid cravings were neither systematically nor widely offered, and follow-up treatment after discharge from a residential facility might be sparse, unaffordable, and punitive, particularly if a client has a relapse, sometimes now called a use incident in an effort to reduce stigma. Although Minnesota has had a much lower incidence of overdose deaths compared to other states, the loss of a loved one is a deep loss, no matter the statistics. As the overdose death numbers rose nationwide during the past decade, individual stories often illuminated the intensity of the national epidemic. When adding up the struggle and pain of each personal story by the number of deaths across the country, the loss to our nation as a whole felt overwhelming and devastating. What an unnecessary accumulation of pain, grief, and tragedy.

Why would this small group of women share such personal, painful stories? It was not because they thought their stories or their children were somehow unique; it was the opposite in fact. The repetition was numbing, the problem demanded change, and each mother hoped her story might help address ineffective treatment protocols, erase stigma, and save lives. No topic related to drug addiction or what they did during that time was off-limits in our conversations. They recalled long periods of time as if caught on a roller coaster of fear, anger, anxiety, and dread. Poor health and strained relationships were the norm. On behalf of their child with substance use disorder, they challenged insurance companies, visited jails, nursed them in withdrawal, transported them to treatment, navigated medical assistance, and found rehabs, detoxes, and doctors. They also lobbied at the state capitol to increase treatment funding and access to harm-reduction protocols; they spoke to high school students, started foundations, and helped other parents on the same journey, whether their own child was still living or not.

For those who were financially, logistically, and emotionally able to provide attention and resources over long periods of time, the ubiquitous pop-psychology critique that they were "enabling" their child's addiction followed them around like a shadow, an additional burden of judgment and disdain.[5] On the flip side, parents who could not afford or otherwise provide that kind of constant attention were criticized as being negligent or ignorant, and thus also stigmatized. Although higher incomes or good insurance plans often provided access to fancier treatment programs, many of these programs were ineffective, particularly for teens. One national study of adolescent-only drug-treatment programs found only modest differences between publicly and privately funded programs, and most all of them met only a medium level of quality indicators.[6] With teen opioid use and related overdose deaths on the rise since the early 2000s, we now know that opioid-addicted adult children from all backgrounds might very likely die.

Historically, mothers have often been blamed for their children's problems, and they have also been socialized to feel a special kind of guilty responsibility if their child developed any kind of social or psychological problem. From the 1950s "refrigerator mothers" who were accused of making their children autistic due to their supposedly cold demeanor, to the 1980s stereotyped "crack moms" who gave birth to "crack babies," these misinformed and misdiagnosed tropes took decades to correct.[7] Regardless of how she mothered, when problems arose among her children, her role and influence was often the most singled out: she was overprotective; not protective enough; too involved; not involved enough.[8] This kind of double bind is a common experience for women and other marginalized groups where "options are reduced to a very few and all of them expose one to penalty, censure, or deprivation."[9] In other words, the well-worn colloquial phrase: you're damned if you do, and damned if you don't. Mothers of children with substance use disorder often found themselves squeezed between the intimate, personal struggles of addiction in their homes and the legal and illegal forces, systems, and institutions outside their homes that rarely seemed life-affirming or caring.

They felt compelled to keep trying and intervening, regardless of the consequences to their own well-being, which fits with one part of the definition of addiction: "People with addiction use substances or *engage in behaviors* that become compulsive and often continue despite harmful consequences."[10] Every mother I have ever met, much less interviewed, would agree that when her child was using, she engaged in compulsive behaviors and continued doing so despite harmful consequences to her health, sanity, and safety. Might fear about her child's active addiction create a parallel addiction to mothering? If so, then mothering addiction has two meanings: one is the experience of mothering a child suffering from addiction; the other is feeling or being perceived by others as being "addicted" to mothering that child. In a generation of parents often referred to as "helicopter parents," I have wondered if the development of hyperalert "helicopter parenting" has had any impact on the long-term outcome of a child's emerging or ongoing substance use issue—did this parenting trend have any impact on drug use prevention, was it neutral, or did it make things worse? For those who criticize these parents, it might appear as if they can't stop helping and intervening, despite the negative personal repercussions amid repeated, ongoing failures. It is more complicated than that, though.

The common pop-psychology term often used for this kind of behavior, "enabling," is connected to another common behavior: codependency, a term first coined in family systems theory. Both words were quickly incorporated into the self-help jargon of the 1980s and became deeply integrated into a multitude of Twelve Step–based peer support groups.[11] Enabling first emerged in the history of codependency during the early years of AA, and at that point it was connected to spousal and family member actions and reactions based on the erratic behavior of an adult, male alcoholic.[12] Melody Beattie, the internationally known self-help author, also from Minnesota, published the most popular book on codependency ever written, *Codependent No More* in 1987. Beattie connected enabling, rescuing, and caretaking and described them all as unhealthy behaviors when doing things for others became engrained as a way of life, a way to be loved through overhelping others, thus centering one's identity on the amount that is done for others. Enabling became therapeutic jargon for these excessive or destructive forms of helping.[13] Something meant to break an unhealthy cycle of caring for loved ones became an easy-out way to criticize caretaking, one of the things parents do best. Although I found a 1985 Hazelden booklet for parents that tried to give the word a positive spin, "Enabling Change," Beattie was read by millions, so the negative concept of enabling embedded itself into the psyche of the Twelve Step culture.[14] One opposing and somehow comforting analysis from the early 1990s argued that the concept of codependency and the enabling that follows was yet another kind of victim-blaming. "The language of codependency blames people, women in particular, for assuming a social role that has previously been viewed as normative and functional. It takes what was once considered healthy, defining it as sick. In the process it fails to acknowledge that change needs to occur at the level of social belief, attitude and expectation."[15] This made more sense to me as I came to know more of these mothers' stories.

Many agreed that if it was enabling, it was done with love in response to fear, not as some kind of unhealthy enmeshment. And nothing really worked anyway. In such circumstances, the dire, pressing need for support from others who understood these mothering disasters led them, more so than fathers, to seek advice from strangers in church basements or in online chat rooms. So very little of whatever herculean actions they attempted, over and over, helped in the long term. Were they addicted to mothering? Were they enabling their children to continue using? Was it, actually, their fault? They had not been trained for this. The patchwork of supports and services for parents navigating their child's often revolving door of active addiction and time in treatment was as hit and miss as finding the right combination of treatment and medication for substance use disorders. This chapter delves into some of the ways that mothers coped, advocated, suffered, and survived the chaos of active addiction.

By the summer of 2012, I felt worn to the bone and desperate to find some kind of solid, time-tested support for my daughter and our family. I had read scores of books about parenting teens, found therapists, tried alternative schools, and had even moved from a neighboring state to Minneapolis to expand the options and opportunities for all of us. What else was out there? What else could we do? During my daughter's teens, much of the well-meaning advice I received from friends and professionals was often neither relevant nor feasible. Despite their kind intentions, I remained isolated and misunderstood. One particularly dark moment, I wondered if I just had to weather the storm of her adolescence and hope she survived. This thought revealed my numb exhaustion, and yet it was a bit too much like surrendering—I wasn't done.

Even while she and I stormed, I tried mightily to change the weather, searching for answers and managing a constant sense of dread about her life and safety. During these years, I worked full time, finished a PhD, and tried to keep some semblance of peace and order in our lives. Madeleine was in a pain I could not reach, an existential, tumultuous battle that began shortly before my divorce from her father and continued for several years after. I felt as if I could never catch up with her, never mind keep her attention on us—or on her own well-being—for very long. She later described these years as being when "we were at each other's throats." That was true.

One especially taxing summer day in 2012, I called a number I found online to ask about a local addiction-related family support group. A gentle voice answered and heard my story. Later that week, I was warmly welcomed by Kathie Simon Frank into a small group of people whose loved ones were in varying stages of remission and recovery from drug addiction. In a brick-and-beige 1970s-era meeting room, I found a group of people who truly understood my experience— without judgment or bewildered sympathy—because they had been or currently were in the very same situation. The self-help books, therapists, and the confounding amount of online advice counted for very little compared to what the ninety-minute, face-to-face meetings offered. Parents of adult children in their thirties and forties were just as troubled as parents of newly drug-using teenagers. Others had family members who had recovered years before, but they attended now to offer camaraderie and support. For everyone, though, repeat traumas were common, as were harrowing stories of homelessness, jail, probation, relapse, overdoses, and all manner of recovery, both short-lived and long-term.

Kathie founded this particular family support meeting in 1997, and she has been there every single week since, barring travel or illness. If it weren't for her tie-dyed socks and Crocs, Kathie, an expert quilter and fiber artist, could just as well have been one of the sweet elderly women I knew from church-basement dinners, so ubiquitous in the Midwest. I felt immediately at ease in her presence. Wise and open-hearted, self-reflective and humble—I found the person I had been searching for.

Nar-Anon Family Groups were founded in 1971 for families and loved ones of people addicted to *illegal* substances. Based on the Twelve Steps and Twelve Traditions followed by Alcoholics Anonymous, Nar-Anon emerged from the more commonly known group, Al-Anon, because of the different circumstances loved ones experienced when the substances of choice were illegal. While a significant percentage of adult Al-Anon members attended because they had experience growing up with an alcoholic parent, Nar-Anon groups were predominantly composed of parents and spouses whose loved ones had a substance use disorder.[16] Both support groups centered around the Twelve Steps and modeled themselves in very much the same way as Alcoholics Anonymous or Narcotics Anonymous meetings.

One psychiatrist I interviewed referred to these meetings simply as affinity groups, which was true, but it's not really something one wants to have affinity with. It was hard and scary to attend those first meetings. But they quickly became a positive experience when, to my surprise, the content we covered was the focus on the well-being of the family members present, not on their loved ones' chaotic drug use and related dramas. Newcomers were encouraged to share the particulars of their current situation by way of introduction, but everyone soon learned this was not the place to air the detailed, ongoing grievances about what addiction wreaked in their lives. The intention was to learn how to be a healthier, more balanced person while loving someone who struggled with substance use disorder. Although some tenets of the Twelve Step program troubled me, I discovered that attending a weekly meeting was grounding and offered moments of calm in the myriad storms I experienced as a witness to chaotic drug use.[17]

Kathie had a previous history with family support groups; her Al-Anon group had long provided help for issues related to other close family members. When she visited her daughter Rachel on the West Coast, she found and attended meetings there. She went to her first Nar-Anon meeting in Seattle. She knew that Rachel was in a troubled marriage and living precariously on the West Coast with an infant daughter, but she wasn't aware of the extent of her drug use. "I was focusing on living as healthy a life as I could. . . . I don't know if I was suspicious of her. I would worry if I wouldn't hear from her for long periods of time. She always seemed pretty put together. I believed this flu thing. Rachel would say she had the flu and I worried about that. I didn't ever put two and two together." Kathie admitted that since drugs were never part of her life—she was scared of them—she never educated herself about them while raising her children. "I chose [not to] read a lot about them. It's not my life. That is an element of denial. I didn't know that flu symptoms were an indication of someone trying to withdraw."[18]

Not long after learning that Rachel was using heroin, Kathie started the Nar-Anon Family Group in St. Paul. For the first five years the weekly meeting remained small, but Kathie was committed to keeping it alive, even on nights when no one arrived. "The word was out, but it wasn't *very* out. We did the best we could to publicize it. We would have between one and five people. In the summer, often I would be the only one who would show up. . . . I'd sit and read the daily reading and wait until seven thirty. If nobody showed up, I'd go home. It was a time for me to center myself."[19]

Even though she had ample stories as a mother of an adult daughter who had struggled with addiction, she rarely mentioned any of that history in the meeting; instead, she modeled for others the program's mission to focus on one's own actions and responses as things arose in all aspects of our daily lives. She shared her own reflections, perspectives, and struggles about the one thing she had control over: herself. For nearly everyone who committed to the ideas set forth in the program, this required a difficult paradigm shift. These parents were accustomed to unrelenting stress, worry, and an overwhelming desire to constantly try to fix their loved one. Yelling, crying, cajoling, and bribing—none of it ever worked. As Kathie explained, the program helped her "turn from a shrieking meanie into a person who could deal with things of great import in a thoughtful way, not denying my emotions but not letting my emotions control me. It allowed me to be in normal relationships with people in healthy ways."

I met two other mothers, Ann Perry and Kim Powers, just a few months later at the same meeting where I had first met Kathie.[20] Both were in emotional tatters from what they had been through over the years with their children, and they, too, arrived thinking the meeting could teach them something about how to "fix" their child's addiction. After a few months driving across the metro area—fairly far from their homes—and now convinced of the support the program offered families, they started a new Nar-Anon Family Group to serve the western suburbs of the Twin Cities. With Kathie's guidance, the group began with about six people but grew quickly, with ample newcomers and regulars filling their suburban YMCA meeting room every week. Mothers vastly outnumbered fathers at almost every meeting, and only a few fathers regularly returned to the group.

One of those regulars was Mike O'Neill, who was referred to the group the first time his teenage son went to treatment. He described his first impressions of these groups to me. "I was stunned at the stuff I heard. Those were real people . . . they were hugging and sharing baked goods and talking about, 'Yes! She got arrested last night. Yay!' Everyone's all excited about someone getting arrested on a felony. I'm like, 'Who *are* these people?'" He kept going each week.

> I started to realize that these were healthy people who had it way worse than I did. I didn't know they had it worse. My son was in trouble, but these were people who'd been dealing with this for a long time and they weren't miserable. They were scared, they were very challenged, they lost sleep at night, but they were getting back to their lives.[21]

Mike openly acknowledged the fact that many more mothers attended than fathers, and he felt badly about this trend. "It just breaks my heart that there are people sitting alone . . . afraid to share because they think they're going to get judged. . . . The dads, I'd love to get more dads to show up because they spend a lot of time very angry, deep in their grief, because they can't fix something. That's a big problem."

The group regularly invited guest speakers to share both professional expertise and personal stories in ways that expanded the meeting beyond the Twelve Step format, with time built in to focus on current issues and education regarding addiction. Initially, the vast majority were parents of adult children who struggled with opioid addiction, so they offered Narcan training as well. Some years later, the rampant return of methamphetamine evened out the numbers of their loved one's drug of choice. Regardless of the drug or the issues of the week, the self-reflection, camaraderie, and humility I encountered among parents in support groups like this was empowering. I always learned something valuable. One of my favorite sayings at the closing of each meeting was, "Take what you like and leave the rest." This gave everyone attending the autonomy and self-respect to grow on their own terms, and it allowed me freedom within the program to filter, contemplate, and imagine a better time for all of us.

More than any support group, though, the fact that my daughter recovered from opioid use disorder was the most powerful factor in my ability to research and write about the epidemic. Had she still been in crisis, I am sure I could not have mustered the strength to proceed. This, combined with the humble introspection I practiced with my support community, freed me to think more broadly about the systemic issues, the underlying, unspoken reasons we came to these rooms each week: the interlocking systems of care and the criminalization of addiction were not working to end this crisis in our communities, much less in our homes. People in meetings often said, "If love could fix this, none of us would be here." We didn't have to question our love—but the Twelve Step model's focus on fixing ourselves, when many of the problems we faced were both socially and politically created, sometimes felt off-kilter to me. In a panicked crisis, in isolation and grief, most people will seek solace and peace in the company of others who share their pain. It was in fact love for our children that called many mothers to question not just themselves, but the policies and protocols that kept the revolving doors of treatment, jail, and relapse spinning on indefinitely. Drug use and addiction are symptoms of a much larger and more formidable intersecting collection of problems. Where families supposedly "fail," law enforcement and other punitive systems fill in the gaps, either with or without the parents' consent.

Depending on who you are and where you live, the options available to parents for emergency help with a child's addiction might not take into account the disease model of addiction, the reason why the addicted brain might commit crimes, or the common prevalence of co-occurring mental health disorders. Linda Berry-Brede was a rural mother who reached out to me via social media to share her story. Although she grew up in the metropolitan area, she raised her five children in and around Kandiyohi, Minnesota, population 491, about ninety miles west of Minneapolis. The largest nearby town is Willmar, where some essential facets of the Minnesota Model for drug and alcohol treatment were developed at the Willmar State Hospital in the late 1940s.[22] She provided one perspective on what it was like to try to manage mental-health disorders and addiction in a rural, small-town setting.

Her son had always struggled with anxiety and depression that was untreated and undiagnosed until young adulthood. At seventeen, he broke his leg and got pain pills. He soon became dependent on Percocet via a doctor's prescription. A shoulder injury a year later insured that his prescriptions were continuously refilled. Eventually, Linda found a pill crusher in the garage; shortly after, he was arrested for selling drugs—marijuana. He went to inpatient treatment at a rural addiction-treatment facility and seemed alright for about a month. Then he was charged with assault for punching the guy his ex-girlfriend had started dating. He was getting a "record" and a reputation in the community. All of this preceded one of her most painful mothering experiences. Her son, then twenty, was living at home temporarily. He was outside with his dad who was burning a brush pile, and fell into it. When his dad pulled him out, he said, "Yeah, I just want to die." He had said as much so many times before in less dramatic situations that they didn't take it as seriously as they probably should have. She carried a lot of guilt about that afterward. It sure seemed like he was "on something," so she tried to calm him. When his brother refused to give him a cigarette and then called him "a spoiled little brat," that got him going. All hell broke loose.

Although he had had similar episodes in the past like this, without drugs in his system, this one frightened her. In this instance, her son hit his brother with a fire poker, attacked his father, and then ran into the woods. When her husband called from the garage to say he thought their son was going to kill him, Linda locked herself in the bathroom, called the county sheriff, whom she knew personally, and said, "I don't know what is wrong with him. I think he is drinking on top of it. We don't know what to do here. He needs some help."[23] The police came, were able to subdue him, and took him to jail.

The next day in the courtroom, Linda was astonished to hear that he was being charged with domestic abuse, terroristic threats, and assault with a deadly weapon. When she called for help, she never imagined these kinds of drastic charges being made against him. He was shocked, too. "He was bawling his head off crying, 'I don't remember it. I don't remember doing any of that. I can't imagine. That's my mom I wouldn't hurt her. . . . I love my mom, I love my dad. I don't know what I am doing here.'" Linda was devastated. "He couldn't remember any of it. My heart was breaking. . . . Although we were scared, we just wanted them to take him and bring him somewhere. To the mental health unit or something. . . . Maybe detox at the most, but mental health mostly."

For decades, the criminalization of drugs and the crimes that often accompany illegal drug use made it ubiquitous and acceptable to treat people with addiction as criminals first, a norm that began with the Harrison Narcotic Act in 1914 that initially targeted doctors for prescribing morphine to patients who had become hooked on it. Throughout the twentieth century, the criminalization approach to drug use became more deeply entrenched in policies and laws with every administration, and more recently is reflected in the ongoing War on Drugs popularized by President Richard Nixon and expanded through the Obama administration.[24] Access to addiction treatment while incarcerated varies widely across the country, with county jails and prisons offering differing amounts of access to support groups like AA and NA, and limited medication availability. Certain Minnesota state prisons now specialize in providing mental-health and addiction-treatment services, but treatment is not mandatory. Ninety percent of Minnesota inmates are diagnosed with substance use disorders (SUD), and the benefits to treatment while incarcerated have been proven, although access to it still appears to be woefully inadequate. Of the 6,500 Minnesota prisoners assessed as needing treatment for SUD, the "department is currently funded to provide treatment to about 1,600" annually.[25] Even though Linda's son was diagnosed with a mental health condition along with substance use disorder, he did not get effective treatment for either while he was incarcerated, so it was not a surprise to her that his crimes continued upon his release. During his first stay at the county jail, Linda and her husband didn't get to visit their son because they were considered "victims" by the state. They begged to not have him charged with anything, but the state charged him with two felonies anyway. He was in jail for months, and afterward his problems just continued.

When Linda recounted this story, her pain was palpable. She described how he was put into a cell with a sex offender and a murderer. Wardens took him off his medication "cold turkey." He was "thrown in the hole umpteen times" for "going berserk."

> He's not really a criminal. He ended up a criminal because of it, but no, he hadn't committed a murder. He didn't do a crime against people, really, it was himself. I was just beside myself the whole time he was in there. I shut it out of my mind because I had to go to work. I was just distraught. Every day I was just sick. I would go to bed and bawl myself to sleep. My husband was feeling a lot of guilt and then sometimes I would just get angry. . . . I went over it so much in my mind. I guess I just talk openly about it to people because I didn't care. I was like, "Yeah, my son has an addiction problem." That is when I joined The Addict's Mom.[26]

The Addict's Mom is a private Facebook group that offers support for mothers of children with drug problems. Social media sites like these have exploded in the past ten years. Spaces for sharing intense personal stories and advice, their easy availability offers thousands of people support and empathy anytime and anywhere they need it. There are pitfalls, of course, when divisive, insensitive politics and stereotypes invade the space, but for the most part, the atmosphere is one of acceptance and understanding. Linda felt empowered finding this group online, isolated as she was in a small, rural community. She spent the four months that her son was in jail forming a working relationship with her son's probation officer, trying to get the charges reduced or dropped and to get him into treatment rather than prison. She even met with the prosecuting attorney.

> I just jumped in there and fought for this kid. "He needs help. Prison is not going to do him any good. Can't you see this? You can save yourself some money by doing something different with him. He needs treatment. Yes, he has been through treatment once but one time probably isn't good. He needs more."

He did end up getting a plea bargain, mostly due to his mom's persistence; he was required to have a chemical dependency evaluation and go to treatment. Linda worked for weeks trying to find a place that was not Twelve Step–based, as her son had not connected with that model during his first stay.

Linda worked for many years at a nonprofit that helped people with severe mental illness care for their homes and perform their daily routines. She remembered she felt on the edge a lot and was hardly able to concentrate, even on simple tasks. Their family property (both home and work space) was about to be foreclosed on. Her marriage was severely strained at the time, too. "My world fell apart."

> I kept thinking, "Other people go through worse things than this. Get it together. Hold it together." . . . I was close to giving everything up and saying, "I can't do this anymore." You get to that point but something keeps you going. . . . I guess I had hope. I would pray and pray and pray. I was a Christian, but I wasn't real sold on the whole idea totally. I thought, what is my other option? I don't have any other option.

The bureaucratic processes took so long that her son was released from jail after four months, with still no spot at the treatment center. His medical assistance took weeks to go through despite her dogged persistence calling back and forth between the facility and the state health department. Linda felt certain that he wouldn't go if he ended up out of jail for too long before going to the rehab.

Three weeks after his release, a bed finally opened up for him. He went. Linda could breathe again. His medical assistance only allocated a thirty-day stay, but at least this treatment center prescribed medications for opioid cravings. He told his mom he felt much better, more clearheaded when he left treatment on medication. Although he connected with the somewhat different model of treatment offered there, its effect did not hold for long. Very few livable-wage jobs existed in their town, and his personal life was in tatters. With each new hurdle, back in the very places those problems first arose, using and selling drugs became more and more attractive. He struggled. At a 2017 sentencing for multiple burglaries, he cried in court and apologized. He was sentenced to forty-five months in prison.

Four tumultuous years later, with her son out of prison and finally on a steady track, Linda has more perspective on what her family experienced. Over the course of several experiences in jails and prisons, the last one ending in 2019, he discovered for himself the situations that exacerbated his already high level of anxiety: parole was better than supervised release, even if it meant he had to serve more time; medical marijuana worked better than any of the psychotropic medications he had ever been prescribed; and, as his mother said, "He finally came across the right people." Linda somehow found a lawyer who kept law enforcement from pinning crimes on him he didn't commit, and then he found an employer in recovery who understood him and hired him. For Linda, her therapist of the past few years has made all the difference for her own mental health and her ability to deal with crises as they arise.

Violating probation for misdemeanor drug offenses, like the presence of drugs in a urine screen or being caught with paraphernalia, could land a person back in jail. Some of the parents I interviewed intentionally had their son or daughter arrested to get them somewhere safer than the streets, though anecdotal stories from jail are not exactly glowing with accounts of safety and caretaking. Even if they didn't directly instigate the arrest, many expressed how they finally slept again if their child was in jail. As hard as it may be to understand, their experiences and seemingly hardened sentiment offer keen insight into how incredibly stressed families become when their loved one is in active drug use.

Kim Powers was one of the mothers who tried to instigate an arrest. She was desperate for any immediate solution that would get her daughter off the streets. She hoped that incarceration or treatment—maybe even both—would provide the time and space her twenty-something, only child needed in order to address her addiction and its related, rapidly accumulating traumas. Once, when Kim's daughter was living on the street and wouldn't agree to treatment—she was violating the terms of her probation by using drugs—Kim took the desperate step of reporting her to her probation officer. Somehow jail seemed safer.

A moment arrived when, while dealing with multiple family stresses simultaneously, she came up with a plan. Her own father had become critically ill and was in the hospital. Kim called her daughter to suggest that she come see her grandfather, who was in a precarious medical situation. Kim prearranged with the security desk to have her picked up by the police at the hospital on the outstanding arrest warrant, when and if she arrived that evening. When her daughter arrived in the hospital room later that evening, Kim was shocked—she had given a fake name at the security desk. She was arrested when she left, though, and Kim remembered feeling very relieved that her daughter would now, for some time at least, be safer in the confines of jail.[27] Parents are never proud of these kinds of actions, even remarking with shock that they barely recognized themselves in that moment, but felt that at the time, it seemed like a better option to use the legal system to try to change their child's behavior when all other private, family efforts had failed. Jail was never the best option for sobriety, however, and these parents hoped that the days their children spent in treatment outnumbered jail time.

When working with insurance companies, state medical assistance, social workers, police, attorneys, judges—even if a mother had access—the age of the child and their willingness to comply, to sign release forms, and to participate in family programming also had an impact on parents. Especially during those days when a bed in treatment is looming on the horizon, the addicted brain can be a fierce and angry opponent. At her urging, Kim's daughter went unwillingly into treatment several times.

> She'd go in—I'd beg her to go in—she'd go in to Fairview, she'd detox for a couple days and then leave. She'd go into [another] treatment [center], she'd stay for two or three days and [then] she was gone. She went to Hazelden twice, stayed for three days. She used heroin in my car in the Hazelden parking lot the night she was going in!

Once in treatment, the adult child often did not allow parents to be included in healthcare discussions and might not even agree to talk to them. The frustration and exhaustion related to getting one's child into treatment and keeping them there happened more than a few times. Among these mothers, eight was the average number of times their children were in drug treatment. Even if their relationships were strained when their child was in jail or rehab, parents took comfort in the fact that, for the moment, as long as they stayed put, they were safe. Death always lurked.

Many of the mothers described health issues of their own that arose from the stress of continued addiction-related crises. Chronic illnesses were common, as were back problems, intestinal issues, anxiety, and depression. Some experienced dangerous breaking points, when even their own lives seemed unbearable. For Kim, that moment occurred when her daughter, her only child, walked out of yet another treatment center. She described her daughter's heroin addiction as "the hardest challenge, the biggest thing that I have ever experienced in my entire life." At her lowest point, she considered ending her own life.

> I almost didn't make it myself. . . . I ended up hospitalized at one point. . . . I tried to commit suicide over this. [She] had left treatment one more time, was back on the street. I just cracked that day. I tried to find her. I was driving around; I was out of my mind. I just knew, she's going to die. I can't outlive her. I don't want to live through losing a child. That's how I felt. That's the craziness that was overcoming me. I can't outlive her. She's going to die.

I began to see a pattern in mothers' persistent efforts on behalf of their children: they were embattled. Caught in a system with her child that often does not serve addiction consistently or humanely, it nevertheless will criticize and chide her, regardless of the mothering she does. When simultaneously navigating emotional crises and institutions like treatment, insurance, and the law, embattled mothering occurs with anxious perseverance in the difficult space between the worst of traditional, apple-pie motherhood and the fierceness of empowered motherhood. Embattled mothering demands persistence beyond reason, patience and introspection, and presence of mind in the midst of chaos, whether that is with her child or with the institutions that must be navigated to try to keep her child alive. Embattled mothering isn't unique to children with substance use disorders. Mothers whose children have different learning styles, abilities, mental-health issues, an LGBTQ+ identity, or who experience racial discrimination might very easily empathize with mothers of children with substance use disorders in their similar challenges to entrenched biases and outdated systems. The pressing need for new policies, protections, and programs would be quite familiar.

The gaps in the overlapping systems currently in place to enforce "drug war" era laws—incarceration for drug addiction and inadequate access to proper, sustained medical care and recovery treatment—have created a battalion of embattled mothers who fight every day to try to keep their addicted child (teen or adult) alive, safe, and hopefully, eventually sober. Many of the mothers I met found themselves caught in a continuous loop of repeated attempts at preservation—of their child's life and their own. Their early experience of mothering, the preservation of a vulnerable life, may have, in fact, gone on for decades. A common sight in family support groups were addled, exhausted parents who had children in their late twenties, thirties, and forties who were still struggling with long-term recovery.

Not everyone found comfort or solace in Twelve Step–based support groups, but by the 2010s, many mothers began sharing personal stories, educating each other and offering advice based on their own painful mistakes and minor successes. Several of them took to social media and other forms of communication and organizing to find affinity communities to work for change. I first met Rose McKinney in 2016 at a one-day conference she co-organized with Know the Truth and Minnesota Adult and Teen Challenge called "From Statistics to Solutions."[28] The purpose of the event was to bring together experts and professionals who work with teens and young adults to collaborate on best practices to address substance abuse prevention and treatment. Rose has a lot of energy and speaks openly about the struggles her son and her family have faced. I saw her as a kindred spirit when it came to relentlessly researching and questioning the status quo.

When her son was in high school, she and her husband noticed some troubling behavior and decided to have him see a doctor. He seemed withdrawn and depressed, and they wondered about possible drug use. She recalled her shock when they learned that the doctor had not ordered a simple urine test for drugs. When they asked about the possibility of drug use, he said, "It is just really tough being a kid these days. He's a good kid. Just get him some counseling." They were completely baffled. Sometime later, during his senior year of high school, her husband discovered aluminum foil with burn marks on it in the car her son drove. He took it to the police who said it was likely heroin, maybe meth.[29] Their son vehemently denied it was his, and around and around they went for the next two years, until he was so deep in his heroin addiction that he had no other option but to begin the revolving door of treatment.

Once substance use disorder has been diagnosed and the teen or adult child is in an inpatient program, the family might be invited to be included in the process. If they attended the family programs, parents found themselves being discussed and dissected as being part of the problem, part of the root cause for the child's addiction. Many parents heard the phrase, "Addiction is a family disease." This vintage trope, much like enabling, has come to mean different things to different audiences, depending on the level of blame and shame being tossed around.[30] In some cases, this may have been true, especially if the parents themselves were in active addiction or if there was emotional, physical, or sexual abuse history in the family. A less fraught but more common meaning was that the family's dysfunctional behavior patterns caused or created circumstances that led to the onset of addiction. Another gentler interpretation of the slogan was that addiction has a negative impact on the whole family, therefore it is a family problem to solve. Although this idea made it easier to conclude that the addicted person brought the chaos of the disease to the family, it ended up blaming them for their disease, which also seemed cruel. Pre-drug use personality and mental health issues such as anxiety, depression, creativity, sensitivity, and self-esteem were also often cited as why or how a child might have had a propensity toward substance use—and this, finally, seemed to take some of the onus off blaming them for the troubles the family experienced.

For Rose, however, mothering had been going well prior to her son's addiction. When he began using drugs, she couldn't see why she and her husband were seen as *a reason* for why he was using drugs.

> Truly, we're *not* perfect, but up until that point of junior and senior high school [we had] a good relationship, and things had been going well. Where the communication dysfunction happened was in [his] drug-induced state. So, no, we were not at our best at all. That was not our main operating style. Even in the Al-Anon world—many positive things to say about that—but, okay, work on *yourself*? I have a crisis over here! I have someone who needs help! I have someone that doesn't realize he needs help, that could die. . . . What I really need is to get my kid in treatment, help my kid stay in treatment, and help him be successful.

Rose's frustration with the whole experience of parenting a teenager who grew into a young adult with substance use disorder led her to create a blog called Our Young Addicts, where she first wrote under the moniker Midwestern Mama.[31] She collected resources, personal experiences, and advice from both parents and professionals as a resource to both find and share information freely. "I knew we weren't the only ones going through it."

After one time in a Twelve Step–based program, followed by a return to drug use, her son was adamant about not going to another one. Her desire to help him find a different type of treatment led to even more frustration. "You look up Minnesota and you get some place in California, and you Google 'non-12 step' [programs] and you get some place in Florida that is a Twelve Step. You've got to be kidding me!" Rose knew that her public relations background and her own business acumen could help address needs specific to teenagers and young adults. The one-day conference she organized for parents, social workers, and mental health and addiction professionals, "From Statistics to Solutions," has been a success for five years in a row and continues to adapt to the changing needs of the community.

Language around addiction has changed so quickly in the past few years that Rose decided to change the name of her organization from Our Young Addicts to OYA to take the focus off the word "addict." When she first came up with the name, her intention was to claim the word "addict" in an effort to destigmatize it and detach negativity from the word by acknowledging that all people with substance use disorders are someone's child. Rose wanted her website to be a place where everyone felt welcome and to continue to be a relevant support resource for families, so she adapted the name to simply OYA.

After experiencing ongoing struggles, parents who continued to help their child were frequently told to not let them come home, to cut off all resources, and to detach. Sometimes the phrase "with love" was added. When applied to families experiencing a loved one with an opioid addiction, this kind of thinking has had devastating, unintended consequences. Many treatment centers have family programs and support groups for loved ones where parents struggle to accept the well-worn truisms—practice "tough love," "detach with love," "cut the addict out of your life," and other "letting go" maxims of pop psychology.[32] If parents did eventually follow some of this advice, it was usually only after having been broken down to the point of depletion, feeling they had no other choice. Ongoing emotional and physical exhaustion often set the stage for such actions. While it might initially sound reasonable for parents to set an obvious boundary of "if you use drugs in our house, you have to leave," following through on this advice when opioids were involved had their child's *possible death* attached as a consequence.

The advice to "detach and let go" was often directly connected to another common trope: the addicted loved ones just needed to "hit rock bottom," and then surely they would stop using. An explanation of what it meant to hit bottom was addressed in the famous Alcoholics Anonymous text known as *The Big Book*. "Why all this insistence that every A.A. must hit bottom first? The answer is that few people will sincerely try to practice the A.A. program unless they have hit bottom."[33] Once AA had become better known nationally between the first printing in 1939 and its subsequent editions, the organization realized the need to "raise the bottom" for others whose drinking had not yet become so problematic as to destroy their lives.[34] By sharing their own drinking histories, they could map what they saw as its inevitable course toward more severe consequences. The concept of rock bottom was meant initially to help people who might be on their way toward severe alcoholism, a scared-straight kind of notion that might help someone become aware of the deteriorating, progressive nature of their disease before it is too late. "Following every spree, he would say to himself, 'Maybe those A.A.s were right . . .' After a few such experiences, often years before the onset of extreme difficulties, he would return to us convinced. He had hit bottom as truly as any of us." Referencing the alcoholic's drug of choice, they argue, "John Barleycorn had become our best advocate."[35] This tied in with another common phrase used in Twelve Step programs: a person's addiction had to "run its course." But with pain pills, stronger heroin, and now fentanyl, a sudden death by overdose can often occur well before someone has even realized the aggressive power of their addiction.

For many of the mothers I interviewed, "hitting rock bottom" was anathema and a sorry excuse to stop helping when all else continued to fail those suffering from opioid addiction. For Janie Colford, waiting for her son's rock bottom was not an option she was willing to entertain. While living off and on at home, trying to go to college, relapsing, and trying both treatment and medication, by age twenty-six he had been in treatment eleven times. Janie didn't care how much time it took for him to heal; she was committed to helping him. When her sister lost her son to a heroin overdose, the tragedy galvanized for Janie what had just been a hunch before her nephew's death. "I believe that rock bottom is death, and why would you wait until that happened? I know that that's not what other people believe and that's fine. To me, I'll do what I need to do to convince him to get treatment if I think things are out of control, or when things [do] get out of control."[36]

Janie Colford was a longtime board member and volunteer at the Steve Rummler Hope Network, the organization where I first learned about Narcan but not about the history of harm reduction. I realized later that this is akin to learning about condoms but not knowing the term "safe sex." Nevertheless, the mix of Minnesota Model treatment, medications for opioid cravings, access to Narcan, and outreach to other families characterized what she and many other mothers juggled with their children. Leveraging their interpersonal skills and professional networks to decrease overdose deaths by changing laws was the next step.

In the winter of 2013, I met Lexi Reed Holtum, then the executive director of the Steve Rummler Hope Network, an organization founded by Steve's parents, Judy and Bill Rummler, following their son's overdose death in 2011. Lexi was Steve's fiancée at the time of his death. She had been with him through his struggles with an opioid addiction that began with a prescription for back pain years prior. A few months after we had first met, she invited me to attend a lobbying day to support legislation that came to be known as Steve's Law. Similar to other laws being introduced across the country, the purpose was to increase training and access to the opioid antidote naloxone for the police and the general public. When administered via nasal spray or intramuscular injection before a person completely stops breathing, naloxone can reverse the depressive effect opioids have on the person's respiratory and central nervous systems—it can bring the dying person back to life.[37] I was thoroughly amazed by the power of this drug and frustrated that I had never heard of it. The bill they helped craft also offered limited legal "Good Samaritan" protections for drug users who called 911 during a drug overdose.[38]

Although I vote and write emails to my elected representatives, actually meeting face-to-face with legislators about a particular topic had never been part of my civic life. Nervously, on a cold but sunny April morning, I made my way to the state capitol in St. Paul, not sure who I was meeting or exactly what I would be doing that day. As

I entered the building, I recognized Lexi among a group of women, so I walked over and started to introduce myself. Before I could say more than my name, five or six of them surrounded me in a group hug and looked sympathetically at me. Then one asked, kindly but directly, "Who have you lost, Amy?" I took a breath, a little startled by the question. Then I noticed they were wearing purple ribbons and big buttons with smiling faces on their lapels, and many were holding photographs. In an instant I realized that most of these women had probably lost a child to an opioid overdose. My daughter was alive, at least as far as I knew. Swirling around me that day was the importance and immediacy of the task at hand, combined with a dark yet legitimate fear about the futures of our living children.

Although I was momentarily overcome by both their warm welcome and the collective enormity of their losses, time was of the essence, and we had a task to accomplish: that day we were to visit as many of the state legislators as possible before an upcoming vote on the bill. I was quickly paired up with a mother named Michon Jenkin who lost her daughter Ashley to an overdose the summer before.[39] As we fanned out in pairs, moving from office to office—sometimes meeting legislators, sometimes just their staff—the power of these mothers' stories to affect social policy became abundantly clear. As the day progressed, I thought of other movements of women in the past who marched and advocated for change: nineteenth- and twentieth-century suffragists, Women Strike for Peace, and Mothers Against Drunk Driving.[40] Besides the half a dozen mothers I met that week, I was introduced to people who work in public health, methadone clinics, recovery advocacy organizations, and treatment facilities. Over the coming months and years, one story would lead to the next, but right then, these women caught my attention. Bound by the familiar deaths of their children and self-educated about opioids, they were determined to change minds, laws, and policies.

Winding up and down staircases, along corridors, and through offices filled with staffers, Michon and I got to know each other a little bit. Each time she told the story of her daughter's death, the legislators were visibly moved; some even teared up. One rotely tried to argue, "Since law enforcement was against it . . . blah, blah, blah." But when he heard about the circumstances of Ashley's death, his meager law-and-order argument crumbled under the power of Michon's bereaved yet completely logical reasoning. Was public access to an antidote overdose drug really that problematic? After spending the day with her and the others, I wondered how anyone could be against a lifesaving antidote being more available to the police and the public.

A few days later in the senate chamber, I sat with these mothers in the gallery above the chamber to witness the bill being passed unanimously. The senate version of the bill, # SF1900, was sponsored by Senator Chris Eaton, herself a mother who had lost her daughter Ariel, twenty-three, to a heroin overdose in 2007. The house version was sponsored by GOP Representative Dave Baker of Willmar, whose son Dan, twenty-five, died of an overdose in 2011.[41] Both were outspoken about the deaths of their children and continued to be involved in legislation related to the opioid epidemic, including an effort to put a penny tax on every opioid pill prescribed in the state to fund increased access to treatment, harm-reduction efforts, and opioid abuse education across the state. That second bill did not pass as envisioned; a swarm of pharmaceutical lobbyists descended on St. Paul and used antitaxation sentiment to fuel objections. The funding to address the crisis in Minnesota would come from the state's general fund.[42]

Mothers engaging in activism on behalf of their children is nothing new in U.S. history, and it may seem similar to groups like Mothers Against Drunk Driving, but it was more than that. They worked against deeply ingrained stigmas about people who use drugs, their deceased children among them, as they went from office to office at the St. Paul capitol building. Their privileged status as white, suburban mothers worked as a kind of shock force—definitely not who most legislators expected would be discussing drug overdoses, the intimate stories of young adult children who died alone in cars, bedrooms, and public restrooms. Their work was altruistic, meant for anyone who might need access to an overdose antidote—from grandma on her pain meds to street outreach workers to harm-reduction organizations in both urban and rural communities. With the tools of social media at their fingertips, they spoke publicly, lobbied for legislation, and founded organizations to address the impact that opioid addiction was having on their communities. Their personal mission was driven by the hope that speaking out might prevent the loss of more lives, so that other families might not have to experience what they did. For others, the organizing became a way to do something constructive when they had no control over their child's current drug-use status or in the face of powerlessness at not being able to have prevented their child's death.

Star Selleck was one of the mothers I met on the Steve's Law lobbying day. She admitted sadly that her education about heroin addiction began with her son Ian's fatal overdose in September 2009. "I realize how ignorant I was at the time that Ian started. I didn't realize how serious it was." She found him on the kitchen floor after coming home in the early evening from dinner with a friend. "When I called 911, the first responder was a policeman who had known Ian since he was very young. They chatted lots. They knew each other. They would sit and talk, [so it] was very hard on that officer to walk in and see Ian [on the floor]. I looked at him and I said, 'He needs Narcan.' He looked at me and said, 'Star, I don't carry Narcan. I can't do that.'"[43] That was when her advocacy began.

Through the Steve Rummler Hope Foundation, Star found an outlet to respond in some small way to the missed opportunity to save her son. She trained others how to administer Narcan. She kept extra kits in her home for emergencies. "If there was a panic, an emergency—a parent that was just finding out—I had people come to my house, all different times, just hurting mothers. . . . I would teach them and send them on to moms' groups." Star became known in her suburban community as someone to call when opioid use was discovered in a family. She admitted that sometimes her work felt like too little, too late, but tried to remember who Ian was in the big picture, over the course of his short life, what he had been like early on.

> You had to talk to Ian about everything; he was way ahead of everybody else. He said, "Mom, did you ever try pot?" At, let's just say, eight or nine. I thought, "Ian is the type of kid you cannot lie to because he will figure out a way [to find out]." I said, "You know Ian, I did try it in college. Then I realized the type of major I had and what I was going to do in life, that I couldn't really keep that up. I couldn't be serious about studying or doing anything with my life and do that, too. So, yeah, I tried it."

She went on to explain to him that once she had even ended up in a very dangerous situation. "My roommate and I drove the wrong way down a one-way street. So, I'm trying to pass on to you mistakes that I made because I don't want the same mistakes to happen to you." Ian's wise reply surprised her. "I don't think that is the way it works. I think each generation has to work it out for themselves." Star smiled at me. "Nobody gets a child like Ian to parent. He just stopped me cold there."

Grappling with what causes addiction or what it "looks like" can be a bitter and difficult experience. While it is changing slowly, most of society still sees drug addiction as a moral failure, or among the more generous, it *begins* as a bad choice—that particular child *decided* to try that particular drug. When caring for their own addicted child, though, most mothers experienced addiction not as a moral failure but as a brain disease, a chronic illness, and a fearsome affliction.

Even the mothers with medical training whom I interviewed admitted they lacked the knowledge needed to find the most effective treatment, believing as so many others do that the abstinence-based model was the best or only way to find long-term sobriety. Even though she was a nurse, Lori Lewis did not understand opioid addiction well enough to explore all of the options for her son. Lori and her husband Monte have four children. When they were small, she ran a home day-care until her two older children, Ryan and Jenna, were school-aged. After they went off to school, she studied to become a nurse, keeping late hours while working and parenting. She attributed both of her professions as directly related to her tendency to be open with her children about health, sex, and drugs. Despite their busy work and school schedules, she and Monte were very involved in their children's lives. As the children got older, their home became a place where school friends liked to hang out.

One evening when a high school friend was over, the kids started talking about health class, where most of what was covered related to sexually transmitted diseases and not birth control. To the embarrassment of the kids, Lori chimed in, "You need to wear condoms. You want to make sure you are ready. You don't know what is going to happen in the heat of the moment." She recalled that her son Ryan's friend turned beet red, and he started laughing. Lori asked him, "'What is so funny? Do you guys not talk about this at your house?' He is like, 'No, that is why I love being over here!'" When their older two children began driving and going to parties, they reiterated their commitment to safety over disciplinary consequences. "We always told the kids, 'Don't worry about the consequences about something. If you are somewhere and you are drinking, and you don't feel safe, I don't care if you are in Duluth, I don't care, we will get you a ride home. Always reach out to us.' But kids, they don't."[44]

When Ryan was a junior in high school, he began smoking marijuana heavily, and after a few serious incidents, they sent him to a thirty-day outpatient treatment center where he could continue his schoolwork. He completed it, and Lori recalled his senior year as being "really uneventful" in terms of drug or alcohol problems. Creative, sensitive, and caring, Ryan was a self-taught musician and a photographer—he took his friends' formal senior portraits. Things were better. As so many parents tend to do—that is, hope—they figured his substance use problems were solved.

Then around age twenty, in 2012, Ryan sank into a depression and hinted at suicide. His girlfriend called Lori, and she jumped into action. Lab tests revealed that he had narcotics in his system. She then discovered that he had absconded with the pain pills she had been prescribed for a back surgery months prior. "Quite frankly, at that time I didn't understand heroin. I didn't understand the disease of addiction. I didn't realize how severe this was. I wish to God somebody would have said to me—honestly, all these counselors—at Hazelden— he's at one of the best places! I wish they would have said, 'If your son doesn't find recovery, it's not if [he] dies, it is when.'" Lori was an attentive mother, with no reason to think that how she had helped and cared for her troubled son was a problem, because it wasn't. She consistently made informed, healthy decisions, but what she didn't know was that she lacked essential facts about the powerful nature of opioid addiction. And at that time, the health professionals caring for her son never directly addressed the dangers with her.

For many parents—Baby Boomers to Generation X—reconciling their own coming-of-age experiences with drug use and addiction with their later experiences parenting a child with addiction is often fraught with misunderstanding, stereotypes, and misperceptions they had about what was currently happening right in front of them. Opioid pain pills were not available by prescription outside hospital settings until 1996, and heroin users were perceived as being on the margins of society, at best. A kind of cognitive dissonance ensued: this didn't look like the heroin addiction they had heard of or knew of, mostly decades before. Yet here it was in the form of prescription pills found in their very homes. And when it became hard to access pills, then to their great shock, heroin and used syringes appeared in the bedrooms of their teens and young adults, mostly using alone, where no one could keep an eye on their safety. Experimenting with drugs and alcohol was definitely on the radar of these two generations of parents raising teens, but the use of opioids took it to an entirely new level of crisis.

Like Lori, most of the mothers began by abiding the recommendations and remedies provided by professionals and authority figures. Yet once they had become more deeply immersed in and confident with their knowledge and experience of addiction, and after having been tested by the structural challenges and failures at treatment, many of them couldn't take it anymore. Besides the common feeling that "everything happens on a Friday afternoon," entire weekends could be spent hoping their child made it through the next few days alive. When that precious call came saying a bed was available, they hoped against hope that the small window of agreement by their child to go to rehab was still cracked open even a little by Monday, or Thursday, or even ten days later. Among the mothers and fathers I met, this cycle repeated itself an average of six to eight times.

Not long after Ryan's second time in treatment, Lori found a syringe in his laundry basket. Ryan had switched to heroin. He was living at home, but not home right then, so she left immediately to track him down and take him directly to the hospital. While waiting in the ER, Ryan began to go into withdrawals; the doctor wanted to discharge him anyway. She went to him and said, "If you discharge my son here, he will probably die, and I will hold you responsible. I don't care what you have to do." They talked to him and put him on a seventy-two-hour hold. "I had left [the hospital] because he was so irate and upset. [Later] I get a call from my husband. They are discharging him anyway. I couldn't believe it." At this moment, Lori knew more than the medical professionals—the authorities—making this decision. She knew the danger that faced him again when he was discharged so quickly and without medication to help his withdrawals.

She returned to the hospital to work out a plan with a sympathetic social worker. The best option for her son turned out to be inpatient treatment, which was not available for more than two weeks. For mothers in this crisis, the next heroin high could mean the death of her child. Two weeks is an eternity. He would surely use again, and as soon as possible, to stop the sickness that withdrawal brings.

Lori's experience with the ER discharging Ryan was common among the mothers I interviewed. When their adult child, either overdosing or in withdrawal, was admitted to the emergency room, they were usually discharged within a few hours, with no follow-up care for detox, treatment, or safe housing. "Treat 'em and street 'em" is what one doctor quipped, acknowledging the danger and disservice of this practice. Some hospitals have begun to change their protocol when it comes to nonfatal drug overdoses. This practice has slowly begun to change in hospitals around the country, especially in places where higher numbers of people overdose. Emergency rooms in Minnesota are beginning to provide Narcan and information about treatment choices.[45]

Lori's son Ryan never did find treatment that worked, despite his attempts to quit using opioids. He went to treatment six times in two years. On July 10, 2014, Ryan Lewis, aged twenty-three, passed away from a heroin overdose at a sober house in St. Paul. He had been in treatment at Hazelden just three days before his death. Lori's anger at Hazelden was justifiable. In his treatment file, every single counselor, psychologist, and psychiatrist wrote: "Is at high risk for relapse if discharged." She was not aware at the time that there were places that treated opioid dependence differently. She saw Hazelden as the best of the best, as many parents do.

On one of his returns there, he was temporarily put on Suboxone (buprenorphine/naloxone), a medication that stops cravings and blocks opioid receptors.[46] Ryan told his mom he felt so much better on that drug—his cravings were gone. But when he was discharged from Hazelden, they took him off of Suboxone and said he should instead have a monthly injection of Vivitrol (naltrexone).[47] At the time, most sober living homes didn't allow residents to be on methadone or Suboxone, including Hazelden's sober houses in St. Paul. Lori asked how he would get the monthly shot. The medical staff suggested she could do it, since she was a nurse. She remembered asking, "Do you know anything about Vivitrol? If I give this to my son while he is actively using, he could overdose and die. . . . You have to do a urine test first. I don't have a urine test at my home."

She decided to send her son to their family clinic to get a urine test and have them inject the medication. Ryan came home angry and frustrated. The clinic wouldn't do it—they didn't know what it was. All of this runaround was so that he could live in a sober home. It perplexed and saddened me to learn that Ryan ended up being referred to Valhalla Place, a specialized group of clinics in the metro area that offers methadone dispensing, Suboxone prescriptions, counseling, drug tests, and other services. He got his Vivitrol shots there a couple of times. This very clinic could have prescribed Ryan the one drug, Suboxone, that had successfully relieved him of his cravings, but none of the sober homes at the time would allow residents to be on it or on methadone. Ryan did not last long on Vivitrol. He overdosed within a couple of months and had to be hospitalized. Back he went to Hazelden. He asked his dad if he would ever get better. The cycle continued until his fatal overdose.

Within a year of Ryan's death, Lori began speaking publicly about heroin addiction at high school assemblies, on local radio programs, and at other community forums, but only in places where they would let her speak openly and frankly about what happened. A couple of area high schools turned down her offer to speak, explaining that they didn't have a heroin or pill problem. She was astonished that they did not want their students to be warned with a real story. Six months after Ryan's death, Lori was quoted in a local community newspaper. "In the end, we couldn't protect our son. No one chooses to become addicted. The person chooses to use that first time but the drug chooses them. We need to recognize this and support people who suffer from this disease. These drugs are a tweet, a text, a Facebook message away. We have to work together as a team or we're not going to win."[48]

Whenever asked, she will always speak, fueled by both anger and resolve to see the system change. At our interview nearly two years after Ryan's passing, Lori said, "I'm at the point now where my grief is turning into frustration. . . . A lot of this was preventable. . . . I don't think he had enough support and tools in the places that are supposed to be renowned. There are so many errors. . . . Ryan was failed by the healthcare system as well. There are a lot of things that I think we can change. When I share my story, I am getting change to happen." Six years after Ryan's death, Lori continues to be active in parent support groups, and people in her community continue to approach her in grocery stores and other places to share their memories of Ryan. Many people miss and remember him.

Embattled mothering has its limits. Mothers moved from exhaustion to rage to despair only to have the whole cycle begin again. Wave after wave of living in crisis takes a physical and psychological toll on parents, and if the child is still living, an overwhelming, empty feeling of loss hangs around. It is not as concrete as death. For mothers whose children died, their grief had processes and supports; although it doesn't go away, the finality of death, its cause and resolution, marks something all humans experience—there are ways to move on. For parents who remain caught in the using-recovery-relapse loop with their grown child, the pain of their losses becomes difficult to explain, much less resolve.

Simultaneously trying to prevent and prepare for a child's death by opioid overdose was common among these embattled mothers. Psychologist Pauline Boss's concept of ambiguous loss, used in her book by the same name, fits precisely the many experiences shared with me about mothering addiction. Examples of ambiguous loss include the kinds of grief related to a missing loved one (missing-in-action military is one example), an autistic child, or a family member with dementia. The lost person may remain unaccounted for over some years or forever; but even without the body to grieve over, psychologically it counts as a very real loss. "The only way to live with ambiguous loss is to hold two opposing ideas in your mind at the same time. . . . It is not part of our culture, however. We like finite answers. You're either dead or you're alive. You're either here or you're gone."[49]

The experience of having a loved one "lost to addiction" fits perfectly with ambiguous loss—it is a condition that has a hope for recovery attached. Someday her child will "return." The addiction has "taken over," many of them will say. The mothers I interviewed seemed capable of persisting in this middle realm with incredible tenacity. Boss notes this ability as an important aspect of the ambiguous loss experience because "to think in a more binary way would involve some denial and lack of truth, so the only truth is that middle way of 'he may be coming back and maybe not.'"[50]

For Janise Holter, the realization that she had to learn to live with the impending-death feeling related to her daughter's heroin addiction occurred at a very precise moment. She was in the hospital at her daughter's bedside. This was the third time she had to be hospitalized for a heroin overdose, and Aly had been on a respirator for three days. No one could predict if she would come out of it this time. Janise realized then she could very likely outlive her daughter. She connected this new feeling to an older one from her childhood. It comforted her then, as it has again many more times during the past eleven years of her daughter's active drug use.

> I grew up in the Vietnam War era, my uncle was in Vietnam, and we lived next door to [a woman] whose son was there. I have very

distinct memories as a child thinking, "I feel sorry for the moms."
All those mothers who had all those children in Vietnam sat in
the same place I sit every day. Not knowing whether or not their
child will survive that day. Why is that comforting? To know that
I am not isolated in being a mother who is on the brink of losing
her child.[51]

The shame and stigma of addiction often isolated families, and although it certainly doesn't have the cultural acceptance that being the
mother of a soldier does, Janise's realization provided a powerful analogy and depth to the idea of embattled mothering. She had learned to
live in the moment and think of other mothers who sat somewhere in
the same situation, be it the present or the past.

Janise grew up in Crystal, a first-ring suburb northwest of Minneapolis. She and her siblings were raised by their Swedish Southern
Baptist mother and atheist German father. Her mother ran a Scandi-
navian craft store, and the entire family worked there. Neither went to
college, and it was never mentioned as an option, but Janise eventually
put herself through college by working, saving, and then paying in full
semester by semester. She eventually became an elementary school
teacher who gravitated toward teaching in charter schools with deep
cultural and community-building missions. Before she studied to be
a teacher, she loved mothering and pursued odd jobs to supplement
the family income. Her two children, Alyson and Andy, brought her
great joy. "I loved being a mother to my kids. I loved it. I was surprised
at how much I loved it." She earned some income by reupholstering
furniture, delivering papers, being a seamstress, but kept caring for
her kids at the center of her life. "I had a kind of a really mellow hippy
existence that I really enjoyed. On my deathbed, when I'm hearkening
back on my life, that will be my period of bliss."

Janise has dealt with more than many. Her daughter Aly, who
struggled with opioids and meth, also battled severe bipolar disorder.
Her son Andy was diagnosed with schizophrenia in his early twenties, and during the worst episode, he spent eighteen months in a
state mental hospital. She learned to navigate laws and court hearings and kept a close eye on his treatment in the mental hospital over
that entire time. Andy now lives in a supervised group-home setting
and sees her once a week. She frequently dealt with these two challenges simultaneously, with occasional lulls from crisis mode when

her daughter was in treatment, jail, or prison, or when her son was steady and content.

An avid reader, a seeker, and a devotee of daily meditation readings, Janise eventually found the most solace in Buddhist teachings. "There, acceptance is everything. Not accepting is all struggle. You accept what it is. You accept that it is yours." Prior to this realization, she could see that she had been "mothering in panic and reacting in panic." She said, "I was not accepting that this is what I got. These are my children."

Embattled as she has been, she somehow has found the strength to thrive in her personal and daily life. She credited her sense of humor for some of this strength. At one point in her interview, she recalled the expression, "when the shit hit the fan." She laughed out loud and said, "Who put *shit* in the fan anyway? Who?" The hard work and the practice of intentionally taking care of herself during these ongoing crises seemed to have paid off. In a comment that connected perfectly with the idea of ambiguous loss, she admitted: "I let myself mourn my losses, mourn the loss of having the kids I thought I would have. . . . There is a good possibility that both of my children will not make it through their twenties. I hope that's not the truth of my life. I will cross that bridge if I come to it. If I come to it, I will cross it and accept it."

A few years after our first interview, that dreaded bridge appeared. Her dear Alyson took her own life on March 24, 2020. She had struggled so long with bipolar disorder, and her substance use disorder compounded it or abated it, depending on what was going on with her mentally. She had been able to achieve sobriety for several months earlier in the year, but there was a cycle to her illness that had a death grip on her mind and body. A couple of days before she died, she impulsively walked out of the workhouse in Hennepin County where she was serving time for violating the terms of her parole related to drug use. The COVID-19 pandemic was in its early weeks. The world felt strange to everyone. Janise was devastated by the news and later came to be grateful for the quiet isolation that the pandemic lockdown created. She truly never fails when it comes to finding a silver lining in even the most painful circumstances.

Several days after Alyson's death, I texted Janise to see how she was doing. She said she was pacing around her house, stalling, doing this and that, but needed to retrieve Aly's cremains. "Do you have someone going with you?" I texted. She replied, "No. I was going to go alone." No way was I letting her do that soul-crushing task by herself! I immediately called and said I would be there shortly. She didn't resist my offer. When she got in the car, we hugged, COVID-be-damned. We made our way on the interstate to an industrial part of St. Paul, where one-story buildings housed all kinds of small industrial businesses and, apparently, a crematorium.

When we walked in, a grandma and two little girls were doing homework in a conference room where various styles of urns were on display shelves. For a second I was puzzled—it sure seemed like an odd place for homeschooling—then I remembered that all schools in the state had just been closed due to the pandemic. The girls smiled at us. I kept my eyes on Janise. Aside from the girls, the place was office-y and yet gently somber. She showed the man at the counter her daughter's birth certificate. He came back with two black shopping bags, one with the box of Aly's ashes and one with her personal belongings. Before we could leave, Janise had to look at an inventory list and then inside the bag to make sure it was all there. I saw the poetry journal Aly kept. The smell of her daughter caused her to step back a bit. "It's all there."

We went to the car, put Aly in the back hatch, and buckled in. Janise started sobbing. We talked in the car for some time. I don't remember anything we said. I just remember being grateful that I listened to my impulse to contact her and then to accompany her on that morning's terrible trip. She had crossed the bridge she spoke of four years earlier. She knew this pain would be different and this loss permanent.

Janise is a seeker and a thinker; her friendship has been a gift to my own self-reflection and growth. These are the sacred spaces outside of the anonymous ones, outside of churches and social media, where the deep work of reconciling our parenting, our children's suffering, and our own place in the world happens. These conversations are so essential to healing and to envisioning a different kind of world for people who struggle with substance use disorders. None of us would ever wish this on anyone, but if we had to endure it, I wanted every one of us to have what I had in that moment.

Years ago, Janise and I smirked in abject agreement at the adage, "It was all part of God's plan." "Seriously?" she demanded. God planned for this or that child to die of an overdose, or this young Black man to spend the rest of his life in prison, or that addiction-afflicted mother's baby to be taken away? While there may be some comfort in the idea of a higher power having a plan for each one of us, this adage more often implied surrendering to something we felt powerless to understand. I worried that it allowed the confused and hopeless to rest on complacency when it comes to solving some of our biggest, most complex, human problems. Even though the disease concept of addiction began to take root in American culture in the twentieth century, judgments about an addicted person's essential moral or spiritual weakness still hold, and they even blame themselves for their addictions. Six months before she passed, Aly posted this on her Facebook page:

> Life for me has never been easy. Not because of my circumstances, but because I made it hard for myself. Why? I never figured it out. Now I've stopped asking why. It really doesn't matter. The only thing I've learned is that there is no bottom to the Rabbit Hole. It goes all the way through to the other side.

Despite advances in medicine, psychology, and evidence-based treatments, so many people continue "paying a price" for mental illness and substance use disorders—in jail, in overdose deaths, in lost lives, in love and time with family. There are too many "rabbit holes," and they are too much like the one from *Alice in Wonderland*, where Alice feels she will be falling forever. Aly ended her post by quoting one of her own poems, "Pieces" from February 2015: "I just wanted my mind to stop racing / I just wanted my thoughts to stop hurting."

What struck me most about these mothers and their families' stories of loss is that, to a person, each one said something akin to, "At least they are out of pain, not suffering any longer." Not having had to face the finality of my own child's death from an overdose, I cannot nor would I ever critique this sentiment or how our minds help us cope through inexplicable grief. But I can say that hearing it so often from dear friends and fellow parents started to make me angry—not at them, but at a system of care in the twenty-first-century United States that couldn't figure out how to truly help them, how to keep them safe and alive. What lessons can we learn from all this loss?

CHAPTER 2

Prognosis Cloudy
Who's to Blame for an Overdose?

On a hot day in early July 2016, I drove out to Minnetonka, a suburb west of my home in Minneapolis, to interview my friend Ann Perry. Severe summer storms the night before had downed power lines, and the sound of humming generators on their cul-de-sac permeated the otherwise bright summer day. Ann was folding clothes when I arrived, and we immediately began talking with an ease you might expect between lifelong friends. Although we had met each other only a few years before, active addiction can pack more drama and tragedy into short time periods than many other illnesses, so on this day in her kitchen, it felt like we had known each other for ages.

As soon as I arrived, Ann told me she had just spoken with a Hennepin County investigator and was surprised because she had already been in touch with one from Anoka County, just northeast of Hennepin. Apparently, a criminal investigation had begun regarding the overdose deaths of several young men in the metro area. One of those men was Ann's thirty-four-year-old son, Spencer. He had died of an opioid-related overdose just three months earlier. It now appeared that law enforcement was going to try to find, apprehend, and charge the drug dealer (or dealers) with third-degree murder.

Ann pondered, "What if they find somebody? Spencer probably would have known this person or asked to buy heroin [from the dealer]."

"Don't you think they are just looking to bust someone on drug charges?" I asked.

"I think they are just going to go as high up the ladder as they can." She paused. "Does it affect me as a mom?"

Ann looked pained by her own question, letting it linger between us, before I replied, "I don't know if it is going to affect you as a mom at all. It's so confusing because it is our child's *addiction*."

Ann said the investigator told her that he "really wants to find this person that made Spencer accessible to his addiction. . . . But there are lots of people who make him accessible." She paused. "I am always so fearful of the public safety people."[1]

"Why? What do you mean?" I don't know why I was surprised by Ann's cynicism, considering how much we both had learned about drugs, law, and the criminal-justice system as it relates to addiction, but I knew her sentiments made sense.

She answered, "Because they are looking for the glory of these big drug busts. I just remember that from when they had the Heroin Town Hall Meeting."

A year or two earlier, when her son Spencer was still alive but struggling mightily with opioids, we met up with each other at a Hennepin County Sheriff Office event billed as a "Heroin Town Hall Meeting" that included law enforcement, some abstinence-based treatment representatives, and Drug Enforcement Agency officials, as well as the state's attorney at the time, Andrew Lugar. Sheriff Rich Stanek was on stage as well, and acted as the emcee, if I remember correctly. Ann had asked the sheriff's staff if she could put flyers out about a new addiction-related family support group, and they reluctantly accommodated her. When she was leaving the meeting that night, she noticed that they had all been dumped in the trash. This stung and came to symbolize for her the frustration and alienation parents of drug users in active addiction experience almost daily. She and her friend Kim Powers, another mother in the group, had gone to the town hall in part to reach out to other parents who might be there. Ann was just starting to feel confident enough as a parent of an addicted child to connect with other parents, and she assumed the sheriff's office and other organizations represented at the meeting that night would be supportive of her efforts to start another suburban Twin Cities family support group. She knew even then about the real possibility of her own child dying, but at that moment she felt more for the other parents in the room, some of whom she knew had already lost children to opioid overdoses. "Remember when the speakers all said we just need to keep our kids in sports and talk around the dining room table? Here sat four front rows of parents with dead children. How insensitive can you get?" I winced because I vividly remembered that the tired, old preventative measure against drug use came from more than one of the featured speakers that night.

"Yeah, have dinner with our children. . . . Our kids aren't in seventh grade anymore. This isn't the D.A.R.E. program."

Ann laughed bluntly, "Well, that didn't work!"[2]

Parents of children with addiction often find themselves in these kinds of murky and bitter situations; it is a dark place, and we just do our best wading through it all, trying to assess and reassess where we have influence and control. Most parents are initially treated by others as though (and also believe themselves that) surely they can wield power over their child's addiction and its related behaviors. They might have a little. They try to believe they have a lot. And since most of us know parents who are not dealing with an addicted child—many of whom think it is simply a matter of influencing and demanding behavioral change—we continue to blame ourselves and look for our shortcomings as parents. Until faced with it firsthand, most people can't understand why "those parents" can't get their child "under control." Other adults make them think they have an abundance of influence, until they don't. And when that happens—that powerlessness over addiction—many parents retreat into feeling shame and stigma themselves: for not having somehow conquered and defeated their child's addiction, for not having been a "good," morally influential parent, like those that have dinner with their kids every night, whoever they are. It doesn't matter if they did all those things the experts recommend—in fact, many of them did; if the addiction progresses to severe substance use disorder, suddenly they are told they don't have any power over their child, and *really never were* able to influence the course of the addiction anyway. It's genetic; it's not. It's a brain disease; it's not. It's family history; it's not. It's not your fault; well it is, actually, your fault. No, it can't be your fault—you did everything you could, you went above and beyond. They are often told that addiction hijacks the brain, that it is physiologically in charge of their child. So, they watch and wait as their son or daughter heads down a well-paved road of dangerous and often law-breaking behavior, whether by simply continuing to use illegal drugs or by committing drug-related crimes. It often feels like a desperate, no-win situation.

Before these addled parents arrive at what later will be explained as the powerlessness of parenting addiction, they are told by drug-abuse educators, community leaders, law enforcement, and other professionals that an effective way to keep their children from using drugs is to engage in wholesome activities: have dinner together every night, get the kids in sports, go to church, and talk about the dangers of drug use. Piloted in 1983 in Los Angeles and used nationwide by 75 percent of schools in the 1990s, the D.A.R.E. (Drug Abuse Resistance Education) program's curriculum was an alliance between the schools, parents, and local police officers who used fear and danger techniques, along with bumper stickers, T-shirts, and other rewards for completing the program. In the late 1980s, one suburban school advertised a dance as a celebration to end a week of drug-awareness education. A common scene at local middle and high schools during drug-awareness weeks in the 1990s and 2000s was when law enforcement parked severely totaled vehicles at the school's entrance in order to scare students about drunk driving. But scaring kids wasn't working. A national study of these campaigns confirmed growing doubts with evidence that such approaches might actually increase substance use among teens.[3] I have no trouble seeing that the opioid epidemic of the past twenty years has defied the drug-abuse prevention platitudes about family meals, safe suburban childhoods, and being from "a good family." Why these ideas persist and continue to plague treatment and health outcomes for people suffering from drug addiction are some of the questions I try to answer, or at the very least expose, with shy Spencer and his tenacious family's story.

Spencer Johnson had a secure and happy childhood. He was born to loving, attentive parents. He attended good schools and had ample access to nature and beautiful wild places, friends, sports, and later, frequent trips to rehab in a state known internationally for its drug-treatment recovery programs. The stereotype of illegal drug users being from broken homes, having absent or abusive parents, and raised in abject poverty still exists, but the recent predominance of white, male opioid users with social and economic privilege, loving parents, and ample access to resources has added a new dimension to the history of drug addiction in the United States.

Spencer's father, Dean Johnson, readily admits that he himself grew up in "Leave It to Beaver Land"—that is, Valparaiso, Indiana.[4] If you didn't know what he has experienced as a result of his son's addiction, it is easy to imagine him comfortably settled in the cozy Indiana town where he grew up or in the wooded suburb west of the Twin Cities where he now lives. He has a gregarious nature, a big smile, and the lean look of an aging high school heartthrob. Dean exudes a happy-go-lucky tenacity, even in the face of great challenges, that can make a person admire his strength or wonder if he's even *seeing* the same things his wife is seeing. And then, in a flash, he might be moved to tears, weeping over his son, someone else's child, or a tender reading shared with fellow support group members.

Spencer's mother, Ann Perry, has a subtle force all her own—she is a quiet, introspective person who questions, considers, and digs into subjects and ideas with an open mind and good humor. She has an easygoing demeanor but maintains a healthy skepticism about life in general, seeking both clarity and understanding, even if the new information exasperates her. In fact, this was how she initially treated her son's addiction: something that needed to be understood. Once she knew enough, she reasoned, she could help him solve his problem.

Ann's early life was scarred by the alcohol addiction of her father, a World War II veteran who was involved in liberating concentration camps, and she attributes some aspects of his alcohol problems to the untreated trauma he experienced during the war. Her father's alcoholism and the impact it had on her childhood skewed her ideas about parenting. When she and Dean first met, she made it clear that she had no intention of having children. Ann experienced a great deal of strife growing up and did not care to repeat any of those childhood scenarios. Her mother had often put her, as the second oldest, in the role of parenting her younger siblings. Ann was more intent on having a career, excelling at her work, and enjoying her life than having children.

Ann and Dean began chatting with each other while standing in line to register for graduate school classes at Southern Illinois University, just outside St. Louis. She was pursuing a master's degree in urban planning. They exchanged phone numbers that day, became friends, and then later roommates, before a romance blossomed. They married in 1977. When Ann was offered a job as a Minnetonka city planner, Minnesota became their new home, and they quickly settled in South Minneapolis. They were married for four years before Ann, at age thirty, changed her mind about motherhood. Their son Spencer was born on July 7, 1981, at a midwife-assisted birth. After his birth, they decided to move closer to one of their jobs and bought a house in Minnetonka.

Spencer attended a family day care on a hobby farm where the children spent hours outside each day. He played T-ball, then baseball, and went to the Y Guide Program with his dad. Ann described his active personality as a lot of "red hair shenanigans," and yet he was also a "very sensitive, shy boy" who didn't like to sleep over at friends' houses. She has no qualms at all concluding that "he had a wonderful childhood." In 1984, Ann and Dean welcomed their daughter Shelley into the family. Ann describes her as a delightful, happy child, and much more outgoing than her big brother. Where he was shy but a risk-taker, Shelley was outgoing and careful. She credits Spencer with teaching her how to take risks and vividly recalled a summer memory at Burntside Lake when he and a friend decided to scale a rock outcropping at the edge of the lake. She tagged along behind them, not wanting to miss out on anything. But once she got up there with them, she thought she was going to fall. Spencer saw her panicking and said, "Follow us, try not to look down. If you do look down just accept that that's your fate." Shelley looked at me wide-eyed and we laughed. "There was rubble and rock at the bottom. It was a terrifying moment that was also a really good growth moment." She paused. "You just confront the next thing ahead and you find the next handhold and the next foothold. . . . You hope you reach the top. We did that obviously. None of us fell to a rocky death."[5]

He wasn't actually dismissive of her safety; in fact, Spencer was also quite protective of his sister. Near their home, they had access to a wetland wildlife refuge and were encouraged to play outside in all seasons. Spencer and some friends had made a fort in the woods. Shelley remembered one fall when they were playing there and heard a buck fight. They were all captivated by it. He saw that it was starting to get dangerous, so Spencer told Shelley, "All right, you have to go inside." He didn't mean go home, because that would mean passing the bucks. Shelley went inside the covered fort and then was indignant. "I did [what he said], and then I'm sitting there, and I'm like, 'Wait a minute! Why does he get to watch?'"

Dean was always struck by the personality differences between his two children. Spencer "was my shadow. He not only looked like me, he walked in my footsteps behind me. I'd turn around and look for him and he'd be right there on my butt. . . . He couldn't talk to people. He was extremely shy. Shelley on the other hand—if some criminal was sitting on a park bench going, 'Hey honey, come over here,' she'd run right over there."

Looking at pictures of Spencer's childhood at her kitchen table, now posted on display boards from his memorial service, Ann glanced tearfully at memories of Slip 'N Slide, wrestling, fishing, homemade Halloween costumes, and their many summers as a family at Camp Van Vac, near Ely, Minnesota. Touching the edges of one, she asked, "How could *this kid* become addicted to heroin?"

When Spencer was approaching junior high, Ann decided to take some time off from full-time work. Her boss had left for another job, and she was no longer happy there. She was also beginning to worry about her son. Like millions of other working mothers in the 1980s, despite a good day care and strong public schools, Ann still worried that her career had a negative impact on her children. She laughed when she shared that she had only lasted three months as a stay-at-home mom. "I was getting crabby" not being stimulated at work, just "rattling around the house" all day. She went back to work again when he began junior high.

At the end of ninth grade, in 1997, Spencer and a friend were caught at school with vodka that Spencer had poured into a pop bottle. He was suspended for two days, and his parents diligently used those two days to meet with a family counselor and have Spencer evaluated by his family doctor for attention deficit hyperactivity disorder. The doctor arranged three weeks of a placebo trial and then determined at the end of it, based on evaluations from teachers and his parents, that some of his school and behavioral issues could be helped with a small dose of Ritalin. Dean explained, "He was diagnosed with ADD . . . he was on Ritalin all through high school. He personally claims that that was what put him down the path [to addiction]. That somehow got him into this habit, even though it's a well-used, monitored, legal medication. He attributed [his addiction] to that."

As Dean recalled, Spencer's attitude about school and life changed in junior high, also part of developmental behavioral changes our society has come to accept, but they wanted to do the right thing—to continue to influence and model positive behavior and good mental health care. Dean vividly remembered one particular visit to a counselor. "This was dismal. The guy was a specialist with adolescents. We go in there and he stands up and . . . his barn door's open!" Spencer started laughing and didn't take the counselor seriously after that moment. After the appointment, he told his parents, "Don't ever force me to go to one of these clowns again." Dean described this as the moment when Spencer "developed a very nasty attitude about anybody who was under the guise of the medical community. He always felt he knew what was in his brain, not some other moron. That was consistent. That developed at an early age."

Spencer used many of the same illegal substances that other kids his age used, and for many years, it played out in very typical teenaged behavior scenarios. When he was sixteen, Spencer and some friends were caught smoking marijuana. Local police approached their car, and when the boys opened the door, smoke billowed out. When Dean shared this story, laughing, his face lit up with a huge smile, imagining the officer's face as he had the boys open the car door. To try to make an impression on them, the police kept the boys a little longer than they had to and then released them. The police notified the school right away, and Spencer was immediately kicked off the varsity baseball team—the one thing he was particularly attached to in school. Ann felt very frustrated by the harshness of this punishment for a teenager, and soon saw the impact of that "consequence" on later problems, like his *increased* drug and alcohol use. "It always impressed me that here [in our community], kids in trouble could not participate in healthy activities." For six months afterward, Spencer went to his first chemical dependency class run by the high school counselor. He later admitted to his parents that he had smoked pot all throughout high school.

Spencer wasn't their only child who struggled with mental health issues. Even though she had always been much more gregarious and outgoing than her brother, Shelley suffered from a sudden and severe bout of depression in ninth grade. Although Ann and Dean's attention was usually focused on both children, for a while during her high school years, Shelley's depression was a major focal point of their parenting concerns. She took an antidepressant that she would later learn, after a suicide attempt in college, was a drug that some early studies suggested might cause suicidal behavior in teenagers.[6] Her medical assessment then changed to a diagnosis of bipolar disorder. She was put on antipsychotics and said she doesn't remember the two years of college when she was on them. Bipolar disorder was also a misdiagnosis. Now in her thirties, she admits, "Looking at it now . . . it was some really hardcore anxiety and puberty stuff. At the time, I agreed with the doctor's prognosis that it was depression . . . [but] ultimately, I became a part of the statistic that antidepressants can make young people even more depressed and suicidal." Despite the setback, Shelley graduated from DePauw University and pursued two more degrees later in theater and education.

While Shelley was still in high school and taking up a lot of her parents' attention (as they all recalled it), the time came for Spencer to go to college. Ann and Dean, who both have master's degrees, pushed him to apply to the University of Minnesota. Ann admitted sheepishly that she probably filled out the application. He got accepted, and he went, but he was very homesick, even though his family was only fifteen miles away. By his sophomore year, he moved off campus with three other friends and, according to Ann, "all they did was party." Spencer's first romantic relationship also happened during his second year of college, with a young woman who had both substance use and mental health issues. Her own parents were unwilling or unable to help her, and soon Ann and Dean began stepping in when she had anxiety attacks, needed to go to the emergency room, or became homeless. Eventually her behavior escalated to the point where they had to ban her from their home, and the relationship with Spencer ended. He dropped out of college not long after meeting the young woman and began working in warehouse and landscaping jobs. Ann wondered in retrospect if it would have been better for him to take some time off before college; she knows they did too much for him by "doing everything we could to keep him in college."

In September 2004, Spencer contracted mono and was prescribed his first dose of Percocet—for a sore throat. Spencer admitted to his mother several years later that he and his girlfriend used to get the prescriptions refilled and would take as many as possible when they partied together. Several years later, he suffered from appendicitis-related abdominal pain and was again prescribed more opiate painkillers. Ann found the label from his first opioid prescription in their house, sometime after Spencer died, and has kept it as a kind of proof or personal record as to when and how Spencer first became addicted.

Sometime after the breakup with his first girlfriend, Spencer met Jamie, a nursing student at the University of Minnesota; they dated for some time before moving in together. She became pregnant, and their son was born in September 2008. By the end of that same year, after Jamie had alerted Spencer's family about Spencer's "weird" behavior, they planned an intervention. Spencer agreed to go to inpatient treatment but insisted it was "only pot." A work friend knowledgeable about treatment programs had recommended to Ann that The

Retreat in Wayzata would be a "good fit" for Spencer and affordable since Spencer had no employer-sponsored insurance and he was too old to qualify for his parents' insurance. Shortly after he was checked in, he went into opioid withdrawal and had to be sent to a detox facility. "We had no idea about the Percocet [or other opiate pain pills], we were very naïve. . . . He came back [from detox] and told us he had taken a couple Suboxone and that's what he had to detox from. We had no clue what that meant." He clearly meant to confuse his parents at this point, or he was taking advantage of their ignorance about opiate addiction. A common "side effect" associated with addiction may include all forms of deception: silence, dismissive comments, minimization of issues, and other retreating and withholding behaviors. And sometimes, parents really don't want to know the whole truth or can't see it, much less imagine that their child is completely lost to an addiction. These two behaviors often work in tandem with each other, and some Twelve Step–based treatment professionals consider this dynamic to be an aspect of addiction as "a family disease."[7] On the other hand, if a family doesn't have access to the professional diagnosis due to patient privacy laws, why would they have assumed opioid addiction?

Even though he hid the truth about his drug of choice, Ann can see now that early on, during his first time in treatment, Spencer really did want to stop using and get on with his life. She found a notepad he used as a diary during those first thirty days. In one of the entries, he was reflective, emotional, and hopeful.

> I need to keep cool and remember how my Dad raised me. No Anger! Keep my dignity always. Talked with Dad about [my] progress. Remember attitude is the biggest problem. He cried at the end of it all. Dean is the best most sensitive person out there. What better model could I ask for. I have been such a little shit in past and could never make up the time or pain I've caused. . . . This experience will always be the biggest turning point in my life.[8]

Spencer also wrote about missing his son, about trying to combat negativity among other residents, and described his vivid dreams—so many took place in the North Woods where their family spent summers, at the cabin and the lake.

When Spencer completed his first inpatient treatment program in March 2009, he moved back in with Jamie and their infant son. He seemed to do well for several months, but by December 2009, Ann recalled that everything had changed again.

> Right before Christmas I remember her [Jamie] calling us to come over to their house because she couldn't wake him up. We couldn't wake him up either. We had no idea. He was probably overdosing. Eventually he came to. Then we brought him to Fairview Chemical Dependency for an evaluation. Of course, he wouldn't let us in. He just thought he should go to outpatient treatment.

Even as a new mother and a partner to a young man struggling with opioid addiction, Jamie successfully graduated from nursing school. Her dream was to be a hospital nurse, but at that time a hiring freeze was under way in Minnesota, so she began applying in other states. In early 2010, Jamie was offered a job in a Montana hospital, and Spencer insisted on going along. He got a job as a landscaper and seemed to be doing pretty well, in spite of repeated visits to Montana clinics and hospitals, a sure sign of doctor shopping for opiate painkillers.

During the next year, Spencer's life began to spin out of control again. Between March 2010 and late November 2011, his parents paid thousands of dollars for Montana emergency room and other urgent care bills. It was around this time that the FDA approved a reformulation of OxyContin to deter what had become a common abuse of the pill—crushing and snorting it.[9] An unintended consequence of the reformulation was that it increased the street value of pain pills, and before long, an ample supply of heroin flooded the market, making it a much cheaper and stronger alternative.[10] Ann believes that this is also most likely the time when Spencer switched from opiate pain pills to heroin.[11]

Spencer's opioid addiction occupied much of 2011. He seemed to be in a constant cycle of pawning Jamie's personal things, doctor shopping in three nearby towns, and asking his parents for money to pay bills, provide him loans, or send cash for other random expenses, most of which were completely fabricated. Ann kept a detailed record, a kind of diary in spreadsheet form, of all the personal issues, needs, and specific amounts of money that Spencer requested, including money they reimbursed to Jamie for her pawned items. Scattered throughout her ledger was evidence of a multitude of lies and mistruths, tall tales, and desperate pleas. Not including medical bills, Ann and Dean reimbursed Jamie and gave Spencer more than $7,000 in cash that year alone, and Ann was sure her records were probably incomplete. In October 2011, Jamie demanded Spencer leave her home by the end of the month. Ann traveled to Montana to get their young son so Jamie could keep working.

For a few weeks after Ann left Montana with her grandson, Spencer remained undecided about leaving the area and used his indecision to try to get more money from his parents, who decided against any more financial help. This forced action on his part and, grudgingly, he returned home to Minnesota in November, where he quickly began pawning and selling *their* personal belongings. Over ten days, and sometimes even twice per day, Spencer pawned a skill saw, lawn mower, snowblower, leaf blower, DVDs, laptop, radar detector, drill, and iPod. When, at the end of this spree, he finally took their car and cash from Dean's wallet, they broke down and called the police on their son. Without access to pills or heroin, he soon went into opioid withdrawal at home and agreed to enter treatment.

The first option they tried was the Salvation Army Adult Rehabilitation Center (ARC) in downtown Minneapolis. He registered on December 16 and then, just before going, decided it "wasn't for him." They found him a spot at The Retreat in Wayzata, Minnesota, again, but a bed would not be available until December 22. That was delayed again by a few more days, a painfully common phenomena at treatment centers; there are often long waiting lists and changes in residents from day to day. On December 26, he finally had a spot at The Retreat. On January 3, he was kicked out for using heroin. He came home and detoxed, again. On January 7, he entered the Salvation Army program and made it thirty days before needing to go to the ER for "stomach pain." He was prescribed Percocet there, too, despite being in a drug treatment program—the physician did not know this important bit of information. When that ran out, he bartered any meager resources he had or borrowed money from other ARC beneficiaries to buy more on the street. On February 19, the day their son went back to live with his mom in Montana, Spencer was kicked out of the Salvation Army program for failing a urine drug screen. Ann and Dean allowed him to come home with an agreement to drug test him. He passed these for a while, but Dean was now convinced that Spencer "routinely cheated them."

It would not be long before drug tests were the least of his problems. In mid-March 2012, Ann typed cryptically and matter-of-factly in her spreadsheet diary:

Drug dealers fronted Spencer 10 grams of heroin ($700) for two former SA [Salvation Army] beneficiaries who were supposed to pay him $1,000. During delivery to SA, Spencer threw the drugs out of the car when cops approached and he never found the drugs.

Spencer was out of control again for another month—pawning their belongings and taking the cash to gamble at the casino for more, only to lose the money (or so he said, but Ann believed he probably used it for drugs). He also began stealing valuables from neighbors, and according to Ann's diary, Dean was able to get all of the items out of the pawnshop. On April 17, they took him to Fairview Detox in Minneapolis, and two days later, he entered the Fairview Lodging Plus program, which he completed. He dealt with his criminal charges that summer and entered a sober house in July, only to relapse two days later, beginning the stealing and using cycle all over again. This spiraling pattern of active addiction, intense drug use, treatment, short periods of relative sobriety, followed by long periods of use and relapse continued for four more years.

Ann related several incidents that highlighted one of her biggest frustrations in confronting Spencer's addiction: finding affordable insurance that would pay for detox and treatment. Spencer's employer in Montana did not offer insurance for employees or subsidize privately obtained insurance. Although Spencer and Jamie had looked for affordable insurance in Montana to pay for treatment for Spencer, he didn't qualify because his income as a landscaper was above the Montana Medicaid limits. When Spencer returned to Minnesota, he was in full-blown addiction and thousands of dollars in debt to Montana health providers. Ann negotiated with the healthcare providers to reduce the hospital debts to an amount that she and Dean were able to pay. Spencer's persistent drug use wiped out any ability he had to pursue his own treatment, diminishing the most basic interaction skills and motivation. Since it was apparent that Spencer could not adequately function to find insurance for himself, Ann decided to take on the task of finding insurance to pay for Spencer's treatment in Minnesota.

The contrast she found between Montana and Minnesota made her particularly grateful for the easier access to resources and programs offered for addiction services in Minnesota. When Spencer returned to Minnesota, he needed to wait three months before he was considered a resident again, and therefore eligible for State of Minnesota healthcare programs. In March 2012, Spencer became eligible for medical assistance. Keeping on top of the changing requirements of the insurance companies at that time was an ongoing challenge. For example, Ann learned that a "Rule 25" chemical use assessment was required for placement in a drug treatment facility in Minnesota. This state-level administrative rule "addresses chemical use assessment, administrative requirements, and appeal and fair hearing rights of the client." Every county, tribe, and "state-contracted Managed Care Organizations are mandated to provide Rule 25 assessments to anyone who requests one, or for whom a chemical use assessment is requested. Clients who meet both clinical and financial requirements are eligible to have treatment paid for by the Consolidated Chemical Dependency Treatment Fund."[12] Despite the generous and expansive nature of the state's treatment options, Ann still found it difficult to find a cost-effective agency that would provide the assessment within the tight time frames she often faced—that small, fragile window of time when Spencer was willing to go to treatment.

After more searching, she discovered that the various treatment facilities had different time requirements regarding the date of an assessment. Some facilities wanted assessments no older than thirty days while others would allow assessments up to forty-five days old. And if this weren't confusing enough, she found that treatment facilities had different length of stay for clients that depended upon the insurance provider. She became very frustrated when one hospital-based program would allow Spencer to stay for only seven days while another allowed him to stay for thirty days, despite the fact that both facilities used the same Rule 25 assessment for him.

One of Ann and Dean's biggest frustrations during this time were the various approaches that treatment facilities and sober homes used toward clients who needed medication for opioid use disorder. For many years, these medications were referred to as medication-assisted treatment (MAT), in that the medication assists with the predominant Minnesota Model recovery method. Some clinical practitioners and researchers have recently started using the term medications for opioid use disorder (MOUD) because it reinforces the evidence that medication is in fact its own treatment and does not necessarily require other behavioral or spiritual practices.[13] Spencer had been prescribed Suboxone early on at a hospital-based program in Minnesota, and yet several nationally recognized treatment facilities that Spencer attended later would not allow him to be on Suboxone or even consider the benefits of it, despite being a client with a pattern of chronic relapse.

When he relapsed on heroin in September 2012, his Suboxone-approved doctor cancelled his prescription and referred him to treatment again. In October, Spencer called asking to discuss his medication treatment. The call was returned by a nurse who told him that he needed to return to treatment and that the doctor would not prescribe medications for him until he completed another treatment program. He returned in November to the emergency room of the same hospital and was moved to a detox facility. He was discharged from detox and went home to get his belongings to take to the next treatment but used heroin while he was home. Later that month, Spencer desperately tried to get an appointment with the same physician and was told by his nurse that the doctor's Suboxone patient limit was full and he was not taking on any more patients.

The following year, Spencer tried inpatient treatment again. He was admitted to Unity Hospital's inpatient treatment program on June 6, 2014, but left against medical advice six days later. His discharge form read "Prognosis: Cloudy" and under "Future Treatment Recommendation," the note said, "Do not readmit the patient for 1 year." After a dozen attempts at treatment, Ann was incensed. "I kept thinking, 'Why isn't this working? What are we doing wrong?' He was on Suboxone. He was probably on Suboxone two years." She, like so many others, knew the familiar treatment and recovery drill regarding MOUD (and by that, they meant Suboxone and methadone): "If you were really serious about your recovery, you should be able to do it without medication."

For what other persistent physical ailment or disease would a licensed health professional write, "Do not admit *patient* for one year," effectively denying them lifesaving treatment? Clearly by this point it was obvious that Spencer could not manage his opioid addiction on his own, but he had learned on the street how to use Suboxone to bridge gaps when he couldn't access treatment or didn't want to use heroin. The choice to not readmit him for a year was at the doctor's discretion, and this one was clearly punitive in nature. When I asked Dr. Mark Willenbring, an addiction medicine psychiatrist in private practice in St. Paul, about this particular situation, he responded that a patient with a high tolerance for opioids who does not do well on buprenorphine (Suboxone) should be referred to a methadone clinic. "There is no justification whatsoever for a one-year period of time when the patient cannot restart. We don't tell people with diabetes or heart disease that they can't get another prescription for their medication for a year if they screw up multiple times. . . . It's moralistic in a harsh way. There appears to be no imperative to treat." He also shared a similar story of a client who was turned away after quickly changing his mind about leaving treatment.

> I recently had one of my patients who took off from [a very prominent local addiction rehab], thinking of going to the bar. Halfway there, he thought better of it and turned back, expecting to be welcomed. Instead, he was discharged immediately, in the middle of the night in the winter. How is it that people feel justified, even prideful, doling out such punishment?[14]

At the time Spencer was looking for housing after treatment, people taking MOUD were more often barred from sober living homes than accepted. This presented a huge challenge for Spencer and his family. Fresh out of inpatient treatment and unemployed, people on MOUD are often unable to secure safe, affordable sober living arrangements. Dean described his outrage at the continued perception in the recovery industry that taking Suboxone or methadone is somehow not being "sober."[15]

> I can't tell you how many philosophical arguments I had with people [who run sober housing]. "Do you take Suboxone?" "No, no, no. We're an abstinence program. We can't have that influence here in our group." I'd go off on a tangent. Why are people putting them on this [medication] and [then] no one out there is tolerating it? One guy says, "I've been in this business thirty

years. We're an abstinence-based house. I can't change. You may
have a valid issue." I always would apologize to people. I'd get so
furious. We'd have the names of forty places, we found two [that
would take him on Suboxone].

The other part of the problem with their son was the issue Dean
described as "exhausting all the options." Of the two places that would
take someone on Suboxone, he was kicked out of both of them for using
heroin. He just couldn't seem to stop, even though he really wanted to.
"He always wanted to go into treatment. He never fought it. Probably
two years ago, we had to throw him out [of the house]. He lived on the
streets for a couple months. Maybe not even that long. He got beat up.
He finally called and said, 'I'm ready to go to treatment.'" His medical
records provide clues to his desperation to quit. In November 2013,
he reported to a doctor: "I want to get my life back, I thought since
I'd been clean for five months I could be with those friends, I screwed
up, I want to be a better father to my son." Seven months later, in June
2014, he repeated this sentiment. His medical record stated, "Spencer
Johnson reports, 'I need to be a better father to my son.'"[16] He wanted
it. He needed it. He just needed more and different kinds of help.

One of the first things loved ones are told in family support groups
is advice known as "The Three Cs": "You didn't cause it. You can't control it. You can't cure it." This doesn't usually go over very well with
newcomers. And neither does Nar-Anon's Step One: "We admitted we
were powerless over the addict, that our lives had become unmanage-
able."[17] Almost everyone who initially arrives at these support groups
comes precisely because they have exhausted their abilities to deal
with their child's addiction on their own; they are looking for the help,
advice, and support of others. Many believe that the more experienced
members will have "answers" about how to "fix" their child's problem,
what to do that will *really* work this time, or how to cope with the sadness and loss that addiction brings to families. Instead, the first thing
they are told is that meetings are not meant for giving advice but only
for sharing "Experience, Strength and Hope."[18]

Learning how to cope with the uncertainty and chaos that active
drug addiction causes is one of the best tools that support groups
have to offer. Oftentimes this meant that parents have to let go of
what they had hoped their child's life would be; all their dreams and
wishes need to be grieved as a real loss. It is no wonder then that

expressions such as "finding serenity" and "detaching with love" resonated with parents who were at the end of their rope. The language
used in Twelve Step programs for loved ones has become part of a
cultural lexicon around how to deal with addictions of all kinds: set
firm boundaries, detach with love, and don't "enable" their addiction
by helping them out of binds.[19]

For years, Ann and Dean went around and around about parenting behaviors that are negatively labeled "enabling" and "rescuing."
Their son was often sick, in dangerous situations, and at great risk
of dying. Was it wrong to pick him up from the side of the highway,
to go find his dealer to pay his debts, to take him home when he's in
withdrawal, to give him money for food? Which action was right and
which was wrong, and in which situation is that *specific* action by his
parents right or wrong? What if Spencer had died when they failed to
help out? How would they look back at that situation or this circum-
stance in which they tried their best or didn't try hard enough? The
likelihood of death by overdose changed the equation, and Ann began
questioning some of those well-worn tenets about how to handle a
loved one's addiction.

> I felt so much judgment from a family member who said, "This
> whole family needs to do tough love. That would solve every-
> thing if we just did tough love." Other people were telling me
> I was doing too much for him. To some degree this is the odd
> thing, especially since he's gone now, doing things to stay close
> to your child—to have a relationship—[that] is so important to
> me. That's what you do as family. But because he has a disease
> like this, you're not supposed to do these things?

Fall 2015 was particularly exasperating, so much so that Ann admitted she finally felt emotionally deadened by Spencer's ongoing heroin
addiction. She made very few notes in her spreadsheet diary the summer before when she spent much of her time alone at their summer
cabin writing, reading, and reflecting.

> As a mom, I just knew that he wasn't going to recover. I had his
> funeral planned out in my head for at least the last year, maybe
> even the last two years. It was tearing Dean and I apart. I felt bad
> as a mother not being able to protect my marriage from that.

Dean felt bad, and I always would get upset with Dean because he was such an enabler. But was that so wrong with what [ultimately] happened?

In late September 2015, Spencer returned to the urgent care clinic where he had gone for his entire childhood to see if he could get help with anxiety that he described as being "out of control," and he also reported chronic insomnia. He was prescribed Klonopin and referred to his mental health providers. No mention was made in this visit of his substance use disorder, except his own admission that he had not been using any illegal drugs. Within a week, he crashed his car, and he continued to be reported for reckless driving, though law enforcement could never find him. He was living at home again. His parents believed then that he was sober, but they were also beginning to notice odd, drug-related behaviors.

In mid-November, Ann wrote in her diary, "Spencer had a terrible bout of throwing up."[20] He was in severe opioid withdrawal. After a few days of ongoing illness and struggling with him, they called the police to their home, and the officer called an ambulance to come to their house when Spencer refused to go to detox on his own. When the paramedics had him in their care, the officer said he would ask the detox facility to keep him as long as they could. Ann and Dean were nearing the end of yet another proverbial rope. As often happens with milder opioid overdoses and withdrawal, the hospital released him at 1:00 a.m. that same night when they considered Spencer's health to be stable. "He called to be picked up, but we refused. Later, a college student called us to say that he had found Spence wandering along the LRT [light rail transit] line. Dean went to pick him up." What had changed between the time he called from the hospital and the time a stranger found him? How easy would it be for a parent to say to a stranger, "Just leave him there?"[21] Ann and Dean struggled mightily with the painful paradoxes of their adult son's addiction. What if he was so unaware that he stepped onto the tracks and was hit by an oncoming train? Now that they knew where he was, how could they not go get him? Ann's frustration remained bitter. Over the next few days, he was still "out of it" and she wrote in the spreadsheet that he missed taking his son to Cub Scouts, and then later that week, he left his son's basketball game early.

Spencer's behavior both angered and devastated his mother. Ultimately, Ann found great solace and support in the family support meeting she attended regularly. She recalled that it was at this point in the fall of 2015, or even earlier that summer, that she dove into her own recovery from her son's addiction and began to let go of the outcome of Spencer's life. She took the Twelve Steps to heart and connected deeply with the spiritual tenets of the program. "I read a lot of Karen Casey's stuff . . . her book, hearing her speak, doing Step work, and I just knew I had to rely on God to get through this."[22] Her voice grew softer as she described her resignation:

> I almost had an epiphany. I remember one day I woke up in the morning and I just felt, I knew it was black and white, there's nothing I can do about this anymore. There's absolutely nothing I can do. It took me a long, long time to get there. Mothering doesn't work, nothing, there's nothing I can do that's stronger than heroin and what it does to my son. The only thing stronger than me is God. I thought if I can survive his death—I knew that's what it was going to be—I'm just going to have to give in to God. I think that's when I felt detached. Then I couldn't do anything. I have to let God do his will with Spencer.

Later that fall, on November 22, in an entry remarkable for its depiction of the insanity families experience with a child in active addiction, Ann wrote:

> Dean and I were on our way to Home Depot and Spence called. Said he was pulled over by the police for an invalid driver's license. Police said they got a call with a report that his car was swerving. When we got there, Spence had [his friend] Evan and his two kids with him. One of the kids was not secured correctly in the car seat. Spencer got a ticket with several violations listed. Dean drove Spencer and Evan to Nordstrom's so Evan could return items—Evan gave Spencer a gift card for returned items. Dean then had to drive Spencer to the pawn shop to get our stuff out and Spencer said he had to give a Black girl the gift card for payment for drugs. Dean refused. They came home and Spencer passed out.[23]

Two days later, despite being pulled over with all the reported violations of reckless driving, Spencer's license was reinstated and he began driving again.

The week of addiction-related crises continued. The day after Thanksgiving, his young son found him lying face down in the bathroom. When he discovered the door locked and knew his dad was inside and not answering, he somehow wiggled the lock open with a Q-tip, then went downstairs to ask his Grandma Ann "why his dad was lying on the bathroom floor." Ann was able to revive Spencer without much effort and then told him he had to leave. While Dean made sure Spencer left the house, Ann drove their grandson around town to distract him. During a heavy snowstorm three days later, Spencer texted her to say he needed to park in the driveway so he wouldn't get hassled by the police. He knew how to get to his mom. Ann wrote in her diary, "My heart was soft and we let him stay the night."[24]

The first three weeks of December were filled with another traffic stop, an arraignment hearing for shoplifting charges, two more withdrawal episodes at home, a chemical dependency evaluation, an appointment with an addiction medicine specialist, and placement on treatment waiting lists. Ann cannot begin to tally the hours and hours she spent to get him placed on waiting lists for treatment, to fill out insurance forms, get approval, wait for a callback, and navigate the bureaucracy of medical assistance benefits. When she pressed Spencer this time about his drug use, he admitted to his parents that for quite some time he had been faking taking his Suboxone by cutting up small pieces of orange paper and putting them under his tongue.

By December 2015, several years into life with a son in active addiction, Ann and Dean had finally exhausted their vast capacity for trying to hide or even trying to make things look "normal" when it came to Spencer. On Christmas Eve, as they always had, extended family members came for dinner after the church service. Ann remembered vividly that Spencer had been "out of it" during the service, "folded over, flat as a pancake in the pew," and must have used again after returning home. "We had the whole family over here, cousins, nieces, nephews . . . Jamie and the kids, everybody was here." Spencer refused to go upstairs, and since his parents couldn't bodily carry him up, they let him just sit there in the living room, with family all around him. Ann noticed the tension in the room and simply stated to everyone,

"This is just what addiction is. This is what they act like." Together, she and Dean decided to not be bothered by it, to just go on with dinner and exchanging presents. Ann recalled, with such tenderness in her voice, "At one point, Spencer was sitting next to my niece, his cousin, and said to her, 'I don't want to be this way at all. I'm so sorry. I just don't want to be this way.'"

A day or so after Christmas, the approved treatment center finally called to say that medical assistance would only pay for four to seven days of treatment. They had to go through the process of finding another program all over again. By this point, Spencer had entered treatment fourteen times; he had successfully completed seven programs and was kicked out of or left the other seven. Although it may seem like a lot of times in treatment, this is not an unusually high number for an opioid use disorder that spans ten years.[25]

Spencer's final time in treatment was at Fairview Recovery Plus, where he entered for the sixth time. Dean visited Spencer as often as he could: "I even cheated a couple of times and just went in until somebody kicked me out." He brought Spencer's son along on Sundays for family visiting day. Dean said Spencer was very optimistic about his recovery this time; Spencer said he had the best counselor ever, and that they encouraged him to get a counseling degree himself to help others with addiction. Dean struggled, wanting to believe that Spencer really believed in his own recovery, but also wondered to himself whether it was just another ruse, the "ultimate in his ability for deception." Ann could not bring herself to visit him there on this, his fourteenth time in treatment. She was completely wrung out. He stayed the entire time and graduated from the program on February 23, 2016.[26] He willingly entered an outpatient treatment program following graduation and told his parents that the program had improved significantly since the last time he attended two years earlier.

As is often the case after finishing an inpatient treatment program, Spencer struggled to find a sober house that had a bed available and also allowed visitors right away. He wanted to see his family regularly, and who could blame him? On March 8, after two weeks living at home again, he moved into a sober house in Columbia Heights, a suburb north of Minneapolis. Ann and Dean didn't initially realize that the man who ran the house was connected to their church and was in recovery himself, but when they did, it seemed like a good omen, a sign of hope for things to come. Within three weeks, Spencer earned his first overnight away from the house and planned to spend it with his son at Ann and Dean's house.

Both of them remembered that they all had a great evening together. The next morning, a Saturday, Spencer said he needed to go to a makeup session at outpatient treatment but would be back by 3:00 p.m. Dean remembered, "Sure enough he came back at three o'clock. . . . I'll tell you, his complexion, everything, all the good signs that you want when you're seeing somebody in recovery. He wasn't broken out with all kinds of crap. He wasn't spooky and talking weird. All of those signs were gone and he spent quality time with his son." Ann agreed. "You could see his personality again, everything coming through." That night before going back to the sober house, Spencer asked Ann to shave his neck because he hadn't been to a barber for a while. "He had his shirt off. He had just taken a shower. . . . I shaved it and I looked all over to see, nothing. He was just my boy again."

Spencer had said he would call the next day. Midafternoon, when Ann and Dean were out in the cul-de-sac where their grandson was riding bikes with the neighborhood kids, the building and grounds director from their church drove up to their house. They knew him fairly well, and he was a good friend of the sober house director, Greg. He said he had something to share, and that they should go inside. Ann thought Spencer had probably been kicked out of the sober house. Instead, he said, "Spencer overdosed. And he died."

Early that morning at the sober house, another resident noticed that the bathroom had been occupied and the door locked for a while. They managed to get it open and discovered Spencer's body. The medical investigator told Ann and Dean that she found him face down in the bathroom with a needle next to his arm, still half full of heroin. This was unusual and a sure sign of a strong dose. She also discovered two more packets of heroin in his wallet and said they would be using those as evidence for a potential drugs charge against a dealer, if that person could be found using DNA. His autopsy concluded that the official cause of death was "mixed fentanyl and heroin toxicity."[27]

The sober house director Greg told Ann and Dean later that day that he had never had a resident die, and many of them were feeling traumatized by it. The house had quickly become a crime scene with tape and police and neighborhood gawkers. They offered to come talk with the residents about Spencer and about what happened, if Greg thought it would help. Ann was particularly worried that his death might upset some to the point of relapse. Greg was grateful for the offer, though he knew it would be hard on everyone, Spencer's family especially. They went the next night, one day after his death, with their daughter Shelley. Ann recalled:

> We told them what we had been through [with Spencer] and told them how we felt and told them how happy Spencer was at the sober house. How thankful he was that he was there. We told them not to give up hope, there's so much hope in recovery. Everybody was crying. This beautiful girl was just sobbing, saying, "I feel so bad for what I put my parents through." So many of them said that. . . . Several of them came up to us afterward and told us how much they liked Spencer, how kind he was and what a compassionate person he was, which was really helpful to me. That's how we brought him up.

After they finished, Ann asked his roommate to show her Spencer's room. She laid down on his bed to see what he would have seen in the room "when he was alive."

Dean remembered feeling like a zombie those first couple of days afterward. With the meeting at the sober house one night, and a meeting with their pastor to plan Spencer's funeral the next, at one point, Dean found himself staring blankly at the ground while outside with their pug, Pee Wee. He remembers he had a strong feeling, and then in his mind he heard the words: "I am not alone, I am finally home." The next morning, the third day after Spencer had passed away, he woke up panicked after a few short hours of sleep, remembering a report he had to write for a client—due that day—for a public hearing the same night. He sat down at the computer, wondering how he could possibly write it, when the phrase, "I am not alone, I am finally home," came back into his mind. "I picked up a piece of paper and in ten minutes a song was there." He was "chomping at the bit" to share this with Ann. She was still sound asleep. He went down and sat in her easy chair by the window to wait.

> I was just looking out the window, and again, not seeing anything, I had my body or my mind filled with a spiritual experience which was not specifically this, it wasn't specifically that. I wasn't seeing something; I wasn't hearing anything. There was exhilaration.

I mean, like fireworks, but I'm not seeing them. My body is slowly getting pumped up. I'm not moving a muscle.

By this time, Ann had come downstairs, and although they were becoming accustomed to seeing each other sitting there looking blankly out the window, Ann asked, "Are you all right?"

I jump up, and I'm going, "This is beautiful!" I'm going, "No, no, no. I'm not some crazy evangelical freak. I don't know what I'm saying." I'm babbling. She's not buying this. She's not coming any closer. . . . "Go over and read that on my desk." She went and saw the music and then she read [the lyrics]. We're hugging each other and crying.

Dean's father had been a piano teacher, and he grew up learning to read music. In the twenty minutes he said it took to write the lyrics, he had also written a tune, a simple musical score, for what he titled "Spencer's Praise," a song that would be sung at Spencer's funeral two weeks later. An excerpt of it reads:

> There was a time I caused no pain,
> There was a time I had no shame.
> How I lived was beyond belief,
> I never meant to cause such grief.
>
> Hallelujah Lord, there are no more tears.
> Hallelujah Lord, You removed our fears.
> Hallelujah Lord, I am not alone.
> Hallelujah Lord, I am finally home.
>
> I only hurt the ones I loved,
> I tried so hard to reach above.
> My life was filled with such despair,
> It wasn't that I didn't care.[28]

Spencer's memorial service was held on April 16, 2016, at their church in Wayzata, Minnesota. For their pastor, deeply saddened by Spencer's loss, this was the fourth opioid-related death that he had officiated in the prior four months. The family decided that they wanted the service to be honest about Spencer's struggle with addiction while also celebrating the goodness in him. "We didn't want Spencer's death to be anything different from [a death by] cancer or diabetes or anything else or have any stigma attached to it. There's no reason not to talk about addiction as part of a celebration of a life event." Four rows of pews were filled with "our people," referring to the sober home residents and dozens of families who attend the support group meeting she founded in 2013. "We didn't want to sugarcoat anything about his life but we wanted to celebrate his life. He had very good parts of his life. He had a wonderful life until addiction took over." High school friends spoke fondly of him, but so did the sober house manager, all while acknowledging the struggles addiction brings. Ann said their decision to conclude the service with everyone saying the Serenity Prayer was "very powerful."

Three months later, sitting in her kitchen, Ann described the tremendous guilt she feels when she attends the family support meeting. "We don't have to deal with the ramifications of heroin use anymore. I can't tell you what that feels like to not have to have that constant worry, that constant pain all the time." Reconciling anger at her son's addiction, the emotional detachment that resulted from the ongoing nature of the illness, and then coming to terms with what or how so-called "enabling" did to hurt or help their only son were just a few of the psychological tussles Ann found herself battling when we met that summer day.

> [I'm] never going to get rid of that feeling. I want to do something, and I get angry. It's the anger. I felt so numb and angry these last three months since he's died. I'm angry because I can't remember the good parts of it. I'm so angry about the addiction parts of him. I felt so numb. I said, "How could this have happened?" Look at those pictures. How could that be, that a disease could be that insidious?

Spencer's loss was sharp and present still, but Ann was beginning to feel unburdened by all the weight that his struggles with addiction added to their daily lives.

Several months later, I went back to their house to interview Dean. Near the end our discussion, Ann arrived home from a blustery winter walk, and the three of us began talking about what we knew about the anonymous drug dealer we first talked about after Spencer's death, now known to us and to the public. Local law enforcement agents had gathered enough evidence to set up an informant-led drug deal that had resulted in the arrest of an African American woman, Beverly Burrell, on May 19, 2016.[29] Burrell, thirty, was charged with five counts of third-degree murder related to the heroin (some of it laced with fentanyl) that she had allegedly sold to each of the men prior to their fatal overdoses.[30] The five men, their ages, and their hometowns, in chronological order of their deaths, were Max Tillitt, twenty-one (September 26, 2015), Eden Prairie; Luke Ronnei, twenty (January 7, 2016), Chanhassen; Dustin Peltier, thirty-one (April 2, 2016), St. Cloud; Spencer Johnson, thirty-four (April 3, 2016), Minnetonka; Nick Pettrick, twenty-nine (April 15, 2016), New Prague.[31] All of them had struggled with opioid addiction, and their personal stories were shared widely in local news outlets. The three of us were surprised by the number of third-degree murder charges and the scope of the investigation.

The case against Burrell spanned four counties and was also the highest number of third-degree murder charges brought against one drug dealer since Minnesota's "drug-induced homicide" law went into effect. The law, passed in 1987, allows prosecutors to criminally charge someone with third-degree murder if they delivered or sold a controlled substance to another person that resulted in an accidental overdose death. One of only twenty states with such laws, Minnesota's cases have increased significantly since 2011, mostly due to the efforts of one Hennepin County prosecutor, Mike Freeman. Although Freeman has said that drug dealers are the "source" of the overdose deaths, prosecuting them for third-degree murder has not resulted in a decrease of opioid-related fatalities, and in fact, despite one dip in 2017, overdose deaths have just continued to rise.[32]

The first trial against Burrell was held over three days in May 2017 and combined the cases of Max Tillitt and Luke Ronnei. For Luke's mother, Colleen, the trial was the culmination of her mission to hold Burrell accountable for the overdose death of her son. Although similar to some of the other mothers I interviewed, she was not only embattled, she had gone to battle for her son against his drug dealer. In local media, she openly described her efforts to catch Burrell herself; she surreptitiously followed her son Luke when he left by car, and once even pursued Burrell in her car across a parking lot, threatening to ram Burrell's car if she sold drugs to her son again.[33] Hennepin County Attorney Mike Freeman, who sought a two-hundred-month sentence for Burrell in Luke's death, said that the third-degree murder charge was designed precisely for cases such as this. "This dealer didn't shoot the heroin into the victim, but they dealt them heroin knowing that it was mixed with other things and it was bad stuff. And it killed them. . . . We need to take these people out of circulation, and that's why we need to be aggressive in charging these cases."[34]

When the trial for Luke Ronnei's and Max Tillitt's death was set, Ann decided to go in order to better understand what might happen when and if Spencer's case ended up in court. She was terribly anxious about the idea of having to attend a murder trial regarding Spencer's death, and she had hoped to keep Spencer's name off public documents. That didn't work. On the first day, a reporter quickly figured out who she was.

Ann's ambivalence about what could be accomplished by charging a drug dealer with third-degree murder remained unchanged from the very first day she learned about the state's intentions a year earlier. She wondered skeptically: Would putting one drug dealer in prison change a drug user's access to his or her drug? Wouldn't it just change the person they purchase drugs from? She also suspected that her years-long experience with Spencer's addiction gave her a different perspective about who is responsible for what in this terrible opioid scourge. She kept acknowledging and reminding herself that Luke and Max were so young, twenty and twenty-one, and that their parents were fairly new to the world of opioid addiction, so perhaps that was why their parents were intent on pursuing a murder conviction.

Sitting behind Beverly Burrell that morning was a group of women—her mother, sister, friends, and other family all packed into a frustratingly small courtroom, side by side with family members of the deceased, local reporters, and others looking to support those involved. That Burrell was a drug dealer was uncontested during the trial. The aim of the county prosecutor was to prove that she was the dealer who sold the deadly dose of heroin to the two young men. Parents took the stand, as did a few friends of the deceased, and the county drug enforcement agent.

At one point, Ann leaned over to me and whispered, "Spence would just die if he knew this was happening." When we simultaneously realized what she had just said, our eyes popped in surprise at each other, and it was hard to stifle a horrified giggle, gallows humor be damned.

But for Ann, it was true. She leaned in and whispered, "Spencer would never blame Beverly for his overdose. He would feel horrible if he knew this was happening." The differences of opinion did not mean that Ann disparaged the desire of the other parents to seek justice in a court of law for the illegal act Burrell committed, rather that she had a different perspective after an exhausting, decade-long relationship with her son's addiction. Spencer knew it was his struggle alone.

Beverly Burrell was found guilty on both counts of third-degree murder and was sentenced to a total of fourteen years in prison in September 2017. At her sentencing, eight victim impact statements were read by family members. The Tillitt family took a different approach to their statements, asking Judge Scoggin for leniency in the prison sentence. Riley Tillitt, who lost his only brother Max, was particularly insistent that Burrell was not the sole cause of his brother's death:

Yes, she sold Max his fatal dose. Had she not, Max likely would have lived longer—he may even be with us today. Yet there are a thousand things that, if changed, may have prolonged Max's life.

Had United Healthcare listened to Max's doctors and recognized the severity of his opioid use disorder, Max may be with us today. If our society viewed substance use disorder as a disease and not some sort of moral failing that deserves criminal prosecution, Max may be with us today.

Ms. Burrell provided the straw that broke the camel's back. She ought to be punished for placing the straw, but not for breaking the back.

No matter how angry I am at Ms. Burrell for supplying the dose that killed my brother, I can't ignore that locking her up for an eternity will change nothing. It won't stop our opioid epidemic. If anything, it might make it worse. It's just economics. With Ms. Burrell off the streets, her clients won't magically quit using—Max never did. Someone else will, rather, someone else already has filled her place as a drug supplier. It's likely that overdoses in Minnesota will continue to grow, regardless of how many people we lock up.[35]

In his sentencing of Beverly Burrell, Judge Scoggin mentioned Riley Tillitt's statement and admitted that he agreed with everything in it, but reminded Burrell and all present that his job was to uphold the law.

There is a great paradox that judges face every day, and this case highlights it probably more than most. On the one hand, we can—we must—deal with the cases that are in front of us. I have to make a decision and impose the penalties that the law requires in a case like this. At the same time, I think Riley Tillitt points out the aggregate effects of the decisions that a whole bunch of judges in a whole bunch of cases make. I don't think they're mutually exclusive. Do I agree that we should treat addiction as a public health epidemic, and that that should be the focus of what society does? Yeah, I absolutely do. But I don't think that that let's someone who feeds that addiction off the hook.[36]

He also acknowledged reading and taking into consideration the reports about the very difficult personal life Burrell has had, expressing some surprise that she would engage in the very activity that has caused so much pain in her family.

I think it would be fair to say that in some ways you have been kicked from pillar to post as you've gone through life. I do know that some of that at least is rooted in the fact that in your own family, in your own personal family, you've had a front row seat to the kinds of battles and misery that addiction causes.

I have to admit that one of the thoughts that I had was that of all the people who would know and understand the kind of pain and misery that the sale of narcotics to an addict cause, that you would be someone who would understand that, maybe more than most of us. I'm not naive, and I know that need to get by, that need to make money blinds us. Makes us ignore a number of things.[37]

Burrell nodded and had to wipe her eyes repeatedly while he was addressing her.[38]

A year later, when she was convicted and then sentenced in Sherburne County, Minnesota, for the death of Dustin Peltier, both the victim impact statements and the judge had a significantly harsher tone. A Minnesota Public Radio story noted that Peltier's father called Burrell "a monster" at her sentencing, and Judge Walter Kaminsky told her, "You made the mess of your own life."[39]

Ann continued to follow news of the upcoming trials, Spencer's especially, with both trepidation and sadness. Her husband Dean wanted nothing to do with them but understood that her interest was one way of processing what happened. "Part of my release, part of my letting go is not wanting anything to do with this. I don't need to read police reports anymore. I don't want the details. It's part of letting go because it can't possibly help me. It might hurt me." He also didn't want his lack of interest to make her feel as if her interest was somehow wrong, either. He recalled his pastor making it clear to both of them soon after Spencer's death that they would have "totally different paths" processing their grief.

Later that summer at their northern Minnesota cabin, Ann and I recorded our conversation about the trial, perched on a rock outcropping that overlooked the lake. "What's going to be interesting if Spencer's case goes to trial is [that] there are going to be significant differences in the description of addiction. That kind of scares me with the press being there. All the ugliness of Spencer's addiction without his goodness will just be out there. I just don't want that to happen."[40] In fact, shortly after she shared this with me, Spencer's cell phone was finally returned to the family, and on it appeared exactly the kind of evidence that confirmed her anxiety about the court revealing the ugliness of his addiction. Ann found text messages he wrote to a friend the day before he died that revealed that Spencer actually knew that the drug he had purchased the day before his death was stronger than usual. Equally surprising to Ann was that Spencer referred to the dealer as "he" and "my dude," not Nicole, as Burrell was known to him. These were the last text messages Spencer wrote before he died.

April 2, 2016 6:13 pm
Spencer: I just od'd and got woke up by a cop
M: Omg. Were you by yourself?
Spencer: Yeah my dude called n fronted me a 40. He said be careful and only do a tiny bit. I did half and woke up to a cop at my window. I'm so lucky. I don't know how I haven't got in any trouble. Wtf this is crazy.
M: No trouble at all?!! Where were you?? What did you say to the cop??

Spencer: I was at 94 and Snelling in St. Paul. The cop woke me
up and took the rig out of my hand. I was out for an hour
and threw up all over myself. Just call me when you can.

M: Okay sorry I'm with my friend rn, but holy shit.

Spencer: That's cool, no rush. Lol pun not intended.

M: So the cop didn't do anything??

Spencer: He wouldn't let me drive so I told him I would take
the light rail home. I had the other half of the bag in my rig
and he took it out of my hand, squirted it on the ground and
threw it back in my car. He made me lock up my car in the
Rainbow parking lot and take the train home. So I waited an
hour and walked back and drove to my parents.

I easily could have gotten a D-dub [DWI] so I'm super
lucky. That's the third run in with the cops in the last 3 days.

I need to stop this shit or I'm really gonna be fucked!!!

M: Jeeze!!! You already had the other half of your bag mixed
up? You need to be careful, for realllll

Spencer: Yeah no shit!!!

M: Good Lord lol

Spencer: Someone's watching over me for sure

M: Yeah for real

The day before he was also texting with another friend, T., and told
her about the same incident. He wrote, "Yeah I'm just lucky I didn't
get in trouble or die. The shit that's going around town is the best I've
ever seen. Everyone's overdosing."[41] When his friend M. texted "what's
up?" the next day at 1:30 p.m., Spencer had already died.

One of the most difficult things for nonusers to understand about
heroin addiction is that regular users often like and seek out the stron-
gest and best high they can find. Over time, the opioid receptors in
the brain adjust to the consistent amount needed to achieve stasis,
so achieving the desired high over and over again requires more and
more of the drug. If one's "memory salience" of the first time using a
drug is strong, the user will often recall that as the high experience he
wants to keep repeating.[42] As one former user described it, "The very
first time I did it, it was like, where have you been all my life? It just felt
wonderful . . . like a warm hug. . . . It went from no big deal to, oh my
gosh, now this is a devastating thing. It's really hard to get out of once
you're in."[43]

Spencer's long struggle and his death by overdose is a painful but extremely common example of how incredibly hard it is to get out from under the grip of an opioid addiction without the right kinds of treatment. The intensity of the cravings and the ease with which one's memory gets triggered about using, even in common everyday situations, can be a fatal combination for a person in early recovery. Spencer moved into New Heights sober living on March 8, 2016. He was in the sober house for less than a month and was clearly still struggling in his recovery, since he began using again shortly after moving in. He passed urine drug screens by using others' clean urine. He knew how to lie convincingly and how to get around the system.

What else could have been done for Spencer? What kind of treatment may have allowed him to finally experience "remission" with his disease? Scientific studies about the success rate of closely monitored, medication-based treatment have shown them to be very successful when used long-term. Yet our system and culture continue to blame the afflicted person, as if they alone can solve their substance use disorder, as if he's just making "bad choices" and perhaps even unable to make any good decisions ever again. Families fall into this thinking, too, and who can blame them? In a country where there are plenty of resources to fix it, but no national resolve to do so, losing hope seems inevitable over time. Ann ultimately came to believe that nothing could be done for Spencer. She and Dean had to find peace in an untenable situation, in a social, political, and medical system that was not working, despite the ongoing, increasing death toll from opioid overdoses. No wonder the familiar Alcoholics Anonymous adage "turn it over to God" had become a common and sadly understandable response to a problem that seemed insurmountable.

As I reflected on Spencer's life, death, and his struggle with opioid addiction, what I questioned was how opioid addiction at its core could be seen as a problem so complex that people suffering from its consequences (users and their loved ones) would resort to believing that solving opioid use disorder actually *requires* some kind of divine intervention. Cultivating faith and hope are essential aspects of being human, yes, but in a country teeming with scientists, therapists, doctors, hospitals, research labs, and treatment centers, how can this particular problem be getting worse instead of better? Why isn't easy access to appropriate and proven medical treatment the norm in our country? The fact that we do not yet have an evidence-based, multifaceted plan to end the current epidemic—one in which we already have solutions and evidence to fix it—further compounds the pain and the continued unnecessary losses experienced by hundreds of family members every day.

For Spencer's sister Shelley, grieving the death of her only sibling in April 2016 took another poignant turn when her private loss paled in comparison to the epic outpouring of sorrow when Minnesota's local hero and internationally beloved musician Prince died of an opioid overdose.[44] "A few weeks after Spencer died, Prince died. Everyone cared so much, and I'm like, 'How do you care so much?' Removed from the immediacy of Spencer's death, I get it, I do, because people become really important culturally. But at the time it was *so hard.*" Opioid-related overdoses and deaths have become so prevalent now in the United States that the overall life expectancy for *all* Americans has decreased as a result.[45] Yet, despite the thousands of people who are daily experiencing private, personal losses due to overdoses, it doesn't have the cultural allure that mourning famous people does—especially cultural icons like Prince. The public responded with an outpouring of sadness and shock that went on for days in Minneapolis and at Prince's Paisley Park compound in Chanhassen, Minnesota. As with many celebrity deaths, the media diligently assembled the highlights of his life, and then we all moved on. Our public grief is evocative, conspicuous, and fleeting. For families who lose someone to an overdose, their private grief remains.

What if there was a way to make visible the losses, fears, and sorrows experienced by everyone over the past twenty years of the opioid epidemic? Very few people would remain untouched by it. If we could see each personal loss as a black armband on the sleeves of our friends, family, neighbors, and coworkers, would we be able to bear the enormity of the loss? Would we be moved to change laws and policies about access to addiction-related medications, treatment protocols, and the failing War on Drugs? Would stigma finally fade? While it is certainly easier to publicly mourn Prince and listen repeatedly to "When Doves Cry," as a nation, we must face the messy complexity and dysfunction of our relationship to pain, drug addiction, and loss. Printed on their son's memorial service program, right under his photo, Ann and Dean acknowledged the importance of ordinary people coming together around tragedy with a quote by Patty Wetterling, another Minnesota mother who experienced the tragic loss of her son to abduction and murder. "When good people pull together amazing things happen. . . . Hope is real. . . . It is a verb. You don't sit back and hope that good things happen. It is all of you showing up."[46]

Three years after I first learned from Ann about the investigation into the prosecution of Beverly Burrell, the last two of the five third-degree murder charges had finally come to court. Everyone knew ahead of time that Burrell planned to plead guilty. Ann invited me to be there with them, and as I stepped off the elevator, I saw family members of all five of the victims gathered in the hallway, chatting quietly before the courtroom opened. I found Ann, Dean, and Shelley talking to the court's victim advocate. Dean commented that it felt like another funeral—"one a *long* time coming." Closure was on everyone's mind. As we filed in, families filled three rows in the gallery area, though fewer attended than at the previous hearings. The parents of Dustin Peltier drove from Belcourt, North Dakota.

The mood was somber. When Burrell came in, she did not make eye contact with anyone. The formalities of the hearing ensued, with a lot of reading of long case numbers by the prosecutor. Once the state made its case and recommended the sentence, Judge Martha Holton Dimick listened as Burrell's attorney Craig Cascarano confirmed out loud with his client everything that happened in both of the drug sales. The court accepted her guilty plea. Burrell sat down, and the family impact statements portion of the hearing began. Since Spencer's family chose not to be taped by the local television station, WCCO, they went first.

I could see both Judge Dimick and Burrell from where I sat. Ann approached the podium. She thanked the court for allowing her to speak and then shared the story of Spencer being prescribed opioids for a sore throat in college, and then again for bouts of appendicitis, after which time his opioid addiction took off. She explained that he switched to heroin when pills were less accessible and that he had been in treatment at least fourteen times. I saw the judge's eyes widen. Burrell shifted in her seat; her attorney looked straight ahead; both faced Ann's back at the podium. Ann's gentle nature and tone of voice belied the power of the story that had distilled in her for the past three years. I don't think anyone expected her to say all that she did. After explaining how his addiction unfolded, she offered a sharp critique of the entire medical and addiction treatment system.

We suffered along with him as his disorder progressed and tried to help him navigate a confusing, stigmatizing, and ever-changing maze of insurance for substance use disorder, recovery programs (many of which were hospital based) that to this day cannot figure out "the gold standard" of treatment, and sober houses that couldn't decide if medically assisted treatment and his use of prescribed Suboxone would violate their principles or values.

I tell you this because I don't hold any blame towards Ms. Burrell for his substance use disorder. My continued anger and disgust are directed towards the healthcare system and pharmaceutical industry that has thus far taken no responsibility for their role.[47]

Ann described the trauma that Ms. Burrell's decision to sell drugs caused—the "rippling impact" it had on so many people—from the residents of the sober house to the investigators, from EMTs to their own Twelve Step family group. She thanked everyone in public service who helped at the scene and afterward. What she learned about addiction in her family support group gave her a deeper understanding of everyone touched by it. She recalled learning that Burrell herself had struggled with addiction in her family and said, "I cannot judge Ms. Burrell for choosing to sell illegal drugs. I don't know what pressures, influences, traumas, or exploitations in her life led her to take the risks associated with selling illegal drugs."

Burrell quickly covered the side of her face with her hand and slumped down a bit in her chair. Ann went on, "If Spencer could speak, he would be the first to forgive Ms. Burrell without any qualms. He always blamed himself for his disorder rather than other people." Burrell wiped her eyes, clearly moved by Ann's testimony. Three years after first saying this to me, Ann's views had not changed. "We know that Ms. Burrell bore no malice towards Spencer and had no intention of participating in his immediate cause of death, although that is a real possibility in her line of work." She concluded:

I forgive Ms. Burrell for her role in Spencer's death and am grateful that she has pled guilty. I trust that if she hasn't already, she will make changes in her life that allow her to find redemption, and compassion and forgiveness for herself in selling Spencer the drugs that caused his immediate death.

In attending the hearings for Spencer's case, I have seen the love and support she receives from her mother and other family members. I hope that their love and support continue while she serves out her prison sentence. She has a powerful story to tell that has the potential for changing others' lives either in prison or out in the world.[48]

When it was Dean's turn to read, he remained seated and handed his statement to the court's victim advocate to read on his behalf. He covered his face while she read. His statement was brief but equally powerful, and reiterated forgiveness and compassion. "He hated his disease and tried gallantly to overcome it. . . . It is ironic that in his darkest times, Beverly was a lifeline. When alternatives for rehab, insurance, and medically assisted treatments were unavailable to Spencer, he turned to the street for the only way he thought he could survive his addiction."[49] Burrell's hand could not contain her tears when Dean described her as a lifeline. The county prosecutor, Mike Radmer, handed a box of tissues to Burrell's attorney to give to her.

Our anxiety and frustration in those times is unexplainable to most and is always with us. My anger at Spencer and Beverly is gone. There is no chance for our own recovery when it is shrouded with anger and anxiety. Our energies are better suited to helping others and fixing the system, which are both still broken.[50]

Judge Dimick smiled as Shelley approached the podium. Her marvelously hip blue and purple hair and her open smiling face took the judge off guard for a brief second. "I am Spencer's sister Shelley. I have arrived at this day with so many emotions and the forefront of those is frustration."[51] She couldn't continue without crying, so she handed the statement to the court's victim advocate and stood beside her while she read it. "I am frustrated at a system that holds only the few at the end of this long chain of problems accountable. Spencer and the four other men involved in these cases paid with their lives, and Ms. Burrell will spend much of her life in a prison system. . . . But what about the other people who provided opioids to my brother. What about the doctors—the people who swore an oath to do no harm—who prescribed it *knowing* Spencer had a huge problem?" Her last line especially resonated with me. "I am frustrated that where we stand today is amid the rubble of the families, and I wonder how many more families will join us."[52] The rubble of the families, indeed. Shelley sat down, exchanging a quick glance with Burrell as she walked past.

It was Nick Petrick's family at the podium now, and they had agreed to be filmed by WCCO. Nick died less than two weeks after Spencer from fentanyl-laced heroin he purchased from Burrell. He overdosed in his car in a Costco parking lot. The camera rolled as his mother and two sisters read their emotional impact statements that focused on their son and brother and on how much they missed him. The older sister spoke openly about Nick's addiction to heroin and read a letter he once wrote when trying to stop using. She said that she visits high schools to talk about her loss and her experience, hoping to have an impact on students. She concluded, "I do not blame Beverly Burrell for Nick's addiction, but I blame her for her greed, turning a profit, and risking lives with no remorse."[53]

When the statements concluded, the judge said she had thought hard about what she could possibly say to the families to convey her sympathy, and after arriving at that speechlessness that so many people feel when faced with tragic and senseless death, she simply said, "I am truly, so very sorry for your loss." She offered the attorneys a chance to make any closing remarks. The county prosecutor had none, but Burrell's lawyer stood up. Craig Cascarano said he had been prepared to be vilified by the families' statements, and so he was stunned to hear Spencer Johnson's family forgive his client. He spoke about how frustrated he had been by the media reports of his client being called the "Angel of Death" and accusing her of having no remorse. He said she was extremely remorseful. She did not know that the heroin she sold to them was laced with fentanyl until the toxicology reports were gathered by him for her criminal defense in the murder charges.

Burrell pled guilty to two counts of third-degree murder and received another twenty-three years, to be served concurrently with the other three sentences of the same duration. As part of the plea, she waived her right to an appeal, and the U.S. Attorney's office agreed they would not pursue her on federal drug charges. Their interest in the case had been part of the delay for the Johnson and Petrick cases.

When the court adjourned, the media and the other families filed out. Burrell and her lawyer were signing papers at the podium. Spencer's family, a close friend of Shelley, and I all remained in the room. Whether it didn't feel right to leave until the judge and lawyers did, or if we all felt pulled to remain seated, quietly absorbing the moment, I am not sure. Whatever the reason, we sat still. Maybe she felt us behind her, but Spencer and his family certainly deserved this moment. Beverly turned her head to the left, looked over her shoulder in Shelley's direction until they made eye contact. She mouthed silently, "I'm sorry. I'm sorry." Shelley's eyes overflowed, and she nodded back.

CHAPTER 3

Prescription for Humility

Opioids and Addiction Medicine

Many of the parents I interviewed for this oral history project mentioned physicians who had touched their lives at some point in their struggle with their child. The same had been true for our family. I sought out doctors because I wanted to learn more about how they approached addiction treatment, which seemed so different from the Minnesota Model and one we had initially and mistakenly assumed was the only way to recover from a substance use disorder. While their personal stories differ, these physicians all practice addiction medicine, whether in clinical or treatment settings. They also generously shared personal experiences and insights about medicine, stigma in their profession, and the meaning of "recovery." Based on their interviews, I began researching and subsequently teaching about the histories of addiction research, pharmacology, and medical innovation that developed prior to and alongside the Minnesota Model. Before reading their individual stories, this chapter requires a bit of historical background about pain and addiction research, about the tensions between science and spirit—that is, between medication and/or abstinence as models of treatment.

Pain is real. Finding relief from it has dogged healers, alchemists, and physicians for as far back as humans have been recording and passing down remedies to alleviate its bothersome and sometimes crippling effects. The pain-relieving chemicals of opium, derived from the poppy plant *Papaver somniferum*, were discovered beginning as long ago as 3400 BCE and spread around the globe from Mesopotamia, China, India, and on to Europe.[1] The sixteenth-century Swiss physician Paracelsus developed an opium-based elixir that he named "laudanum," from the Latin "to praise." The isolation of the active alkaloid morphine in 1804, and then the invention of the hypodermic syringe in 1853, changed medicine, surgery, and pain relief forever. Nothing has ever compared to its effectiveness at blocking pain.

Nineteenth-century efforts to diminish the intensities of opium's properties paradoxically resulted in the development and creation of an even stronger substance. Morphine was more powerful than opium, and when its side effects and addictive properties began to manifest in dangerous and deadly ways, the drug company Bayer employed one of its chemists, Felix Hoffman, to acetylate morphine—that is, add an extra chemical group to it. He hoped to create a drug with fewer side effects than morphine. Instead, the experiment resulted in a substance that worked much more quickly and was nearly twice as strong.[2] Bayer trademarked it as Heroin, from the Greek for "heroic, strong," and in 1895 the company began selling it as an over-the-counter medication, advertised as and believed by physicians as safer than morphine.[3] We know where that eventually led us.

When trying to reconcile how our country got into an even more dangerous place with pain pills, heroin, and even stronger synthetic opioids today, the eerie familiarity of the main players in this century-old history, the physicians and drug makers, can be both maddening and disheartening. The 1995 FDA approval of OxyContin, a slow-release opioid pain pill, was heavily marketed as being safe and nonaddictive to doctors and consumers by profit-driven pharmaceutical companies. Yet since 1999, more than 450,000 Americans have died from opioid-related overdose deaths, with most of these deaths caused by opioid pain pills. Millions more suffer from ongoing opioid use disorders.[4] To understand the many players behind this tragedy, one has to look to the recent political and social history of how Americans deal with pain, and particularly how both conservatives and liberals responded when a free-market healthcare system intersected with a powerfully addictive and aggressively marketed medicine.[5] Although this most recent opioid epidemic has created a dire public health crisis, researchers in the United States have been actively studying drug dependence and addiction since the 1930s.

Addiction research began in 1935 in Lexington, Kentucky, at the first federal facility for drug addiction, known as the Narcotic Farm. Built for the "complete social rehabilitation of America's drug addicts" and jointly run by the Bureau of Prisons and the Public Health Service, the aim of the institution was what historian Nancy Campbell has called nothing less than audacious.[6] The one-thousand-acre campus with lodging, farms, and a research facility was both a prison and a treatment center where patients participated in multiple kinds of treatment: group and individual therapy, religious services, and even as subjects in scientific research. Some arrived voluntarily and others were serving prison terms for drug offenses, but everyone was there for a hard drug addiction. For decades, the Addiction Research Center, located on the premises, was the only research center of its kind dedicated to answering pressing questions about drug addiction, succinctly encapsulated by Campbell: "Why do some drug users become addicted and others do not? What makes addicts willing to sacrifice home, family, and everything they care about for a substance that is obviously killing them? What causes relapse?"[7]

We still don't know definitive answers to all of these questions. We do know that the reward circuitry in our brain, when combined with the opioid receptors on its nerve cells, can create a powerful addiction to and craving for all opioids. In 2016, the National Institute for Drug Addiction estimated that 23 percent of individuals who use heroin develop a heroin addiction, and roughly 21–29 percent of people prescribed opioid pain pills misuse them, with 4–9 percent transitioning to heroin.[8] Even if a person wants to quit, the physical and mental cravings, combined with intense and unpleasant withdrawal symptoms, are often too difficult to handle without significant medical and psychological help.

Drs. Vincent Dole and Marie Nyswander began studying methadone as a maintenance medication for opioid addiction in the 1960s. Both had been working in this new field of addiction research before collaborating and pioneering the use of methadone for people addicted to heroin. Over a multiyear study, Nyswander and Dole discovered that daily low doses of methadone allowed their patients to resume normal, healthy, and functioning lives. The medicine worked to block opioid receptors in the brain, and their subjects no longer craved heroin. By 1967, they had collected data on more than five hundred subjects and built the case in several scholarly articles for the maintenance of narcotic addicts on daily oral doses of methadone, and reported that "once stabilized on methadone they began eating regularly, regained lost weight, attended to their hygiene and ceased being preoccupied with narcotics."[9]

Methadone's evidence-based effectiveness and long-term success worked against it in the morals- and abstinence-focused therapeutic culture that was starting to become known across the country. Despite being tested on a wide variety of former users over several years and, notably, without a need for Twelve Step or therapeutic community-type behavioral and moral interventions, its critics saw it as a "seductive panacea . . . that let the sources of addiction go untreated and lulled a patient into a false sense of normalcy."[10] When methadone clinics were established in inner cities in the 1970s as a way to curb the drug-related crimes of people with heroin addiction, the clinics themselves became sites of racial stigma as well. Methadone was perceived as a treatment of last resort, a drug for the addicted criminal or the hopelessly addicted. The low cost of the treatment came to be associated with people who lacked access to other resources for recovery, and the clinics, heavily monitored and regulated by both the Drug Enforcement Administration and the FDA, were an unappealing and even inaccessible option compared to inpatient drug treatment centers.[11] All of these factors strengthened the idea that going to an abstinence-based, residential treatment program was how people truly recovered from addiction, that using medications for opioid use disorders was somehow a lesser and morally weaker achievement than complete abstinence.

Since the mid- to late twentieth century, the growing popularity and prominence of abstinence-based treatment centers made it seem almost unnecessary to see a family doctor, internist, or psychiatrist for help with a substance use disorder. In fact, if a drug or alcohol problem was addressed at an appointment, primary care physicians were more likely to refer their patients to drug treatment counselors and programs than to offer any expertise of their own, if they had any. A few factors led to this: the burgeoning treatment industry; changes in health insurance coverage; the development and spread of employee assistance programs that linked employees directly with mental health and substance use disorder resources; and the overwhelming success of the self-help movement and its literature.[12] In medical school, physicians were not trained thoroughly, if at all, to even discuss substance use disorders, so when a patient needed this kind of care, contacting a drug treatment center directly became the default, especially when active addiction had escalated into a crisis situation. Thankfully this changed somewhat in the 1990s. Although physicians embody the bridge between science and human suffering, and have created organizations devoted to understanding patient drug and alcohol use since the 1870s, addiction medicine was not accredited as a subspecialty until 1991, when psychiatrists "had the foresight to develop the subspecialty of addiction psychiatry."[13] As of 2014, forty-six one-year accredited fellowships are available across the United States to interested physicians. Despite these gains, this number is small considering the vastness of specialties available in U.S. medical schools.

Indeed, the significance of the Minnesota Model in the state itself is so prevalent that one of the doctors I interviewed referred to Hazelden as "the Vatican" and Alcoholics Anonymous as Minnesota's "state religion."[14] He did not mean this completely sarcastically—the monolithic influence of it in drug abuse treatment programs has been integrated into nearly every treatment center in the United States since the 1950s.[15] All other kinds of treatment, especially medications used for opioid addiction, have had to struggle to be seen as anything less than periphery to the power of the Twelve Steps. Even the commonly used term for prescription medications that treat opioid cravings, medication-assisted treatment (MAT), was a reference to the centrality of Twelve Step–based treatment. The medication was *assisting*; it was not seen as central to recovery. In 1997, the Narcotics Anonymous World Services office addressed this issue in "Bulletin #29," a document that explained their stance on the topic. NA welcomed members who were on "drug replacement programs" to attend meetings, but they were only allowed to share in the meetings if their group chose to allow them to participate. "Our program approaches recovery from addiction through abstinence, cautioning against the substitution of one drug for another. That's our program; it's what we offer the addict who still suffers."[16] The issue has continued to remain contentious in the wider recovery and addiction treatment community. In 2011, William White, the well-known author of *Slaying the Dragon*—a text used widely in addiction counseling education programs to teach the history of abstinence-based alcohol and drug treatment programs—carefully and almost apologetically examined the contentious issue of medication for opioid use disorders among Narcotics Anonymous groups. In a government grant-funded report, he prefaced his findings with this caveat:

> Its purpose is NOT to influence NA's views on these issues, but to help explore ways in which addiction professionals and recovery support specialists can enhance the peer-based recovery support

available to patients in medication-assisted treatment. These are, of course, controversial issues that we (author and reader) are about to explore. What follows is not intended as a final statement, but an invitation to sustained reflection and dialogue from multiple quarters on the question of the best ways of achieving long-term recovery from opioid addiction.[17]

Ultimately, the report reveals how polarizing the issue of medications for opioid use disorders remains in NA and AA circles, even as White attempts to bridge the chasm and make suggestions for cooperation and improvement from both sides. Despite science-based evidence of their efficacy, in some AA and NA circles, the use of medication to control opioid cravings can disqualify a person from participating in their group's leadership roles, claiming full sobriety, or even being considered substance-free. Choosing to keep their medication private, which makes sense if the meetings are helpful, paradoxically puts the person at risk of being dishonest—a character flaw that goes against core tenets of the Twelve Step program. These double standards reinforce a no-win, shame-generating cycle. White's report points out in passive language, such as "it could be argued," that people on medication who are not warmly welcomed in NA groups are at risk of losing out on the therapeutic benefits that the fellowships provide and thus may be more likely to return to using.[18]

One of the earliest questions I had for healthcare and treatment professionals was whether recurring rehab failures and high death rates associated with opioid use disorder might finally cause these two powerful institutions, the medical/scientific community and the spirituality/affinity groups, to collaborate to improve their outcomes. Because substance use disorder is rarely treated as a medical issue, many people fall through the cracks with their physicians. For Twelve Step–based programs, the unwillingness to fully accept people who choose medications for opioid use disorder as being truly sober or "in recovery" is another significant problem. Whether it is stigma or precedent keeping these groups from changing their teachings, it is still troubling. Historically, I can see how the siloed worlds of abstinence-based programs and scientific addiction research came to be, but from a human rights and public health perspective, I still cannot understand why stigma about medications for opioid use disorder persist in so many settings, both institutionally and socially. Such siloing has had deadly and devastating consequences for how "clients" in treatment and "patients" under supervision experienced, succeeded, or failed to control their opioid use disorder.

Surely, we are capable of holding two truths in tandem and maybe even work in cooperation with each other, integrating the best each approach has to offer? What follows are some insights and answers to this question based on the education and, perhaps more powerfully, the lived experiences of physicians who have devoted their careers to healing others and themselves.

Charles Reznikoff, MD

Dr. Charlie Reznikoff was the first doctor to explain to me how medications for treating opioid addiction worked. We first met in 2012 when I had sought out resources and also wondered what I could do to alert other naïve parents like myself to the influx of heroin to Minnesota. He connected me with an opioid task force, an education and outreach foundation, and other healthcare professionals. Several years later, he agreed to share his story at the clinic where he sees his patients.

The addiction medicine clinic where Reznikoff works opened in 1994, after a few years of planning and negotiation with the sprawling Hennepin County hospital. Known for decades in the metro area as HCMC, Hennepin County Medical Center spans six city blocks near downtown Minneapolis just steps from the shadow-casting U.S. Bank Stadium. Although the name has been changed to Hennepin Health, and the neighborhood around it has gentrified somewhat, the clinic continues to serve many low-income patients. The methadone clinic was founded in June 1994 and was organized by a few very determined doctors from Hennepin Faculty Associates, a private, nonprofit medical group of over four hundred physicians. Their initiative, tenacity with their board, and outreach to the community brought the addiction medicine clinic to a neighborhood and patient population who needed it. They first used the only pharmacotherapy available at the time, methadone, and then followed with naltrexone in 1997, disulfiram in 2000, and buprenorphine in 2007. A research division of the clinic has allowed physicians and researchers opportunities to improve services, many of which are community-centered and culturally specific, like the Hmong medication-assisted treatment program, run by Dr. Gavin Bart. One innovation that did not gain traction was a two-year, grant-funded mobile medical unit that would have dispensed medication in neighborhoods where clients lived, with the goal of making medicine more accessible and reducing the chance of missed doses.[19]

The clinic was bustling on the cold January morning when I went to interview Reznikoff. The first thing I noticed when I entered was the crowd of people of every age and ethnicity, waiting in chairs arranged to fit as many clients as possible into a small waiting area. Dr. Reznikoff popped out from a side office to greet me, dressed in snow boots, jeans, and a flannel shirt. Nothing about him commanded authority, but everyone's head turned when he came to find me. We settled into a consulting room just off the waiting room, and he shared his story.

Charlie was born into a medical family—he is the son of a biochemist father and oncologist mother, and grandson of a noted hematologist. Early in life, his mother told him he could either be a priest or a doctor, but he had to have a life of service.[20] His dad was less directive, and Charlie conceded with a smile that his mother would have likely accepted some other career choice. Laughing, he explained to me that by the time he was twelve, being a priest was out, and he began imagining himself as a doctor someday. His older sister, now a mathematician, kept him in line with her intellectual force—correcting his grammar, his logic, and his thinking—and he affectionately attributed his ability to deal with a critical verbal environment to her. His older brother was much like a twin, only ten months older. He was adopted when Charlie's parents thought they couldn't have another child, and then, as is so often the case, they immediately conceived again. He credits his brother for teaching him about humor, art, and music. Charlie reflected that as an adopted but also very close sibling, his brother taught him about the power of genetics but also about the limits of genetics. His brother was more of a risk-taker, but not by much. "Whatever 'dumb' is, I did 95 percent of it and he did 105 percent of it."

Charlie attended public schools in Madison, Wisconsin, and after high school was accepted into a premed-type program at the University of Wisconsin called Medical Scholars. If students maintained a high GPA throughout their undergraduate coursework, they were guaranteed a spot at the University of Wisconsin–Madison Medical School. The program was special in that it allowed students some freedom to explore other academic subjects and not feel so stressed about getting accepted to medical school. Charlie realized the privilege of this situation and believes it set a precedent for his pay-it-forward attitude. He entered medical school knowing he had been given something special and needed to do good things with it. "I had incredible fortune."

During his internal medicine residency rotations at HCMC, a family member of his was struggling with opioid pain pill addiction, so he reached out to an addiction medicine doctor he knew from Madison, Dr. Rich Brown. Shortly after, Charlie signed up for an addiction medicine rotation and loved the patients and the work involved. Two things happened that confirmed addiction medicine as his specialization. One is a fable, as he called it, but the way he told the story also made it seem like a door to his heart opened that day. During his first year of residency, he saw a young Black man with medical issues related to a congenital heart problem. While they were discussing his case, the young man confided that he was a heroin user. Charlie didn't know what to do with that information. He wrapped up the appointment. A couple of days later, as he was walking down a hallway in the hospital, a receptionist's phone rang.

"Yeah, actually yes, he's right here." Then the receptionist looked at Charlie. "Someone just called this phone and asked for you, Charlie."

It was the patient again. He was crying, "I just injected heroin, and I don't know what to do." Charlie could hear people yelling in the background. He didn't know what to tell him, so he told the man to go to the emergency room, which he wasn't sure was the correct advice, but he didn't know what to tell him. By then, a group of people had gathered at the desk, wanting to know what happened on the call. "I told them that a patient that I saw three days ago randomly called this phone number and asked for me and confessed that he had just injected heroin. . . . In some ways that was my vocation calling. . . . That's my future calling. That was a true story."

The second reason he committed to addiction medicine occurred during his year as chief resident, when he got to know Dr. Gavin Bart, an addiction medicine researcher at Hennepin Health. Dr. Bart offered Charlie an opportunity to work in addiction medicine at the methadone clinic as well as on other addiction-related care—a tobacco clinic and a Rice County buprenorphine clinic. He would also work with University of Minnesota medical students.

Besides his career trajectory, I had questions about why methadone was so pigeonholed as a treatment. The stigma that surrounded it confused me early on, and then once I knew more, the racism connected to it frustrated and saddened me. The stark class and racial disparities between suburban drug treatment rehabs and urban methadone clinics made no sense to me if one simply looked at the science of medications for opioid use disorder. But if you take a sociological approach to the geographies and patients at these facilities, it is clear that the long-standing stigma of drug abuse directly correlates with stigma surrounding poverty, systemic racism, and the bootstrap myth that persists in American society.

Charlie laid it out bluntly and honestly. "The demographics of a methadone maintenance clinic—the demographics of heroin twenty years ago—was Black, urban, felons. If you're an affluent, suburban, Caucasian person, the idea of going to a clinic that is highly Black, urban, poor, with some mental health and felonies mixed in—well, racism and classism took over." In other words, methadone treatment itself became conflated with the stigma attached to a particular demographic of heroin users. He likened it to the early days of the HIV/AIDS epidemic. When it became evident that everyone could contract the disease, and not just gay men, attitudes about research, medicine, and prevention efforts became more widespread. The same is true with heroin and opioid pain pill addiction. "People don't understand that methadone reduces death, prolongs life, improves pregnancy outcomes, reduces incarceration, reduces IV drug use, reduces hepatitis C and HIV transmission . . . the medicine helps stabilize [you, because] once you are addicted, you have an incredibly high death rate. Methadone lowers the death rate in that person in a controlled setting." Reznikoff was clearly bothered by the classism and racism inherent to methadone as a treatment, especially when Black Minnesotans have died from opioid overdoses at twice the rate of white Minnesotans. "Opioids absolutely have no racial, gender, or age preference. This is absolutely a democratic addiction, and it is fatal."

Fighting the stigma associated with methadone adds an additional layer of burden on people seeking help for an opioid use disorder. One 2013 study found that when taken together, "experiencing and anticipating prejudice, stereotypes, and discrimination from family and friends, as well as coworkers and employers may undermine mental health and methadone maintenance therapy success among patients in addition to stigma experienced from healthcare workers."[21] Equally angered and saddened by how long we have let the stigma of methadone linger in the African American community, Reznikoff hopes that the large numbers of white people from a different demographic being lost to overdose deaths will focus renewed attention on an evidence-based medical approach to saving everyone's lives. Situated where he is in downtown Minneapolis, he explained, "This is something that has been endemic in the North Minneapolis Black neighborhoods for decades and decades and decades. Now that it is affecting affluent, suburban kids, people are freaking out. I get it. But I roll my eyes at it."

The year he began working at Hennepin Health was exactly when heroin use began quietly emerging as a problem among suburban and small-town white kids.[22] Years before the media started reporting heavily about pill and heroin use among white youth, Reznikoff had been seeing a young patient from Northfield, Minnesota, who found him online as a buprenorphine provider. He drove up to the Minneapolis clinic every month. "He told me stories about a hidden heroin epidemic among teens in Northfield and started bringing other kids with him for appointments, 'like the pied piper of opioids.'"[23] One of the mothers of these Northfield kids, Judi Malecha, lost her son Jake to an overdose in 2007. Though Jake was never a patient of Charlie's, Judi had heard about him. She leveraged the hospital in their town to contract with Charlie for some of his time. He began driving there one day every other week and continues to do so.

The clinic has since moved into a family practice setting in Lonsdale, Minnesota. He smiled when he spoke of this particular clinic and reported that on his most recent day there, he saw twenty-three patients in five hours. "It's incredibly rewarding. . . . Two of my twenty-three patients were using heroin still. The rest were sober. I get drug screens, I check their prescription-monitoring program, but more [than that] I just *know* these patients. I meet with them regularly. One of them just got offered a major promotion at work. These people are really thriving at work and are really happy."

And yet, addiction medicine doctors often report that the social stigma associated with drug users looms just as large among doctors themselves, many of whom can't imagine why someone would want to specialize in and treat such difficult people. The stereotype he described was nearly identical to that described by every other doctor I interviewed, that addiction medicine must involve "a series of emergencies" where doctors have to "deal with people that don't want to be there, whose lives are blowing up, who are lying their pants off." To the contrary, his patients are "people who have accepted that they have a disease, who are working to get back to a relatively normal life, and who are working hard. Most of them are in treatment. We help them get there and help them attempt to have a perfect life. It is really rewarding." He described the long-term, fulfilling doctor–patient relationships he has developed over the past several years, with individual patients he has seen sixty times over eight years, with fifty or more of those visits solid check-ins to report great progress. The other times were what you might expect when managing any kind of long-term health issue; crises arise and doctors help the patient figure out the best course of action. Worries about relapsing, recovery, and other triggers are par for the course, and as such, Reznikoff believes these are best managed under the care of a physician.

Robert Levy, MD

Like Charlie, Robert Levy was also born into medicine: both of his parents were New York psychiatrists. He grew up in Brooklyn and remembers his childhood fondly. "My parents both loved me a lot. They both have their own intricacies and quirks, but really, they were great parents. They gave me too much, but not *way* too much. I went to a private school growing up, and I had great friends." Although he was an only child, his father had been previously widowed. By the time Bob was born, the youngest of his three half sisters was eighteen and headed to college. His mother passed away in March 2016, but his father, in his mid-eighties, now lives in Los Angeles with his third wife. Sharing this, and how great his dad is doing, made him smile and joke, "He married a younger woman—she's in her seventies."[24]

His laugh matches his overall demeanor, and it is easy to imagine him being a physician with whom his patients feel comfortable talking. We met in a conference room at North Memorial Hospital in Minneapolis, adjacent to the primary medicine clinic where he practices. Bob recalled that he wanted to be a doctor for as long as he can remember and persisted with it despite his own parents discouraging him from the profession. "I have a very vivid memory of being in seventh grade, taking biology class in school and thinking, 'This is the first step. I have to do well in biology, so I can do well in high school, so I can do well to get into college, so I can do well to get into medical school.'" He has always liked talking to people, hearing their stories, and helping them. He says this with all sincerity, knowing how cliché it must sound. I believed him.

Levy was equally candid and forthcoming concerning his relationship to addiction medicine and how it came about as one of his areas of specialty. His own anecdotal knowledge of other doctors in the field shows a close correlation between personal experience with addiction (self, family, friends) and an interest in it as a specialization. He has dealt with addiction himself, as a user of fentanyl, and is as open about this as he is emphatic to explain why he always tells people that he had a great childhood. "When people hear you have an addiction, they assume your childhood was terrible. I can say that I was never really bullied. A little bit, but never badly. My parents never abused me. I had a great childhood!" He also says he cannot blame his parents for his addiction, even when they asked him what they did to "screw [him] up." He remembered that his answer to them was, "You know, not everything is about you guys!" He laughed again, and then we dove into his story.

Drinking alcohol and smoking marijuana are often referred to as "gateway" activities on the way to being a hardcore addict, but this assumption has not played out in the interviews I have conducted and doesn't fit with Bob Levy's story either. He smoked pot and drank some alcohol with high school friends, but never got in any trouble over using it and didn't do it in excess. As a student at Carleton College, he quit drinking as much because he wanted to focus on his studies. He remembered one semester when he smoked too much pot and got a B- in a class, his first "low grade," which prompted him to stop that completely as well.

In March of his senior year, he fell and fractured his ankle in several places and vividly remembers that first dose of morphine in the ER. Levy quickly explained that in addiction medicine this kind of moment is referred to as an example of memory salience. "All this anxiety and this tension and this stress in my life all evaporated. It was really miraculous." The physical pain was bad, yes, and abated quickly, but what he remembered most was his chronic anxiety lifting, disappearing, and feeling wonderful for a brief amount of time. "It was an intramuscular injection of morphine. I remember that very, very clearly.

And that, in addiction medicine, is called salience . . . that is a bad sign when someone remembers it very well like that. . . . I remembered it very clearly." Then he repeated again, "It was miraculous." The pain going away was one benefit, but the memory of being free of anxiety stayed with him for much longer.

Due to the multiple fractures, he had to have surgery and went home to New York. He remembers taking a lot of oxycodone for pain relief during his recovery from surgery, but not the euphoric feeling of the first morphine. What he does remember was being more chatty and talkative when he was using it, but nothing more than that. Several "life pain" situations arose when he returned to school—his friends were graduating and leaving, his girlfriend broke up with him, his mother got very sick; he couldn't do much and wasn't "fun to be around." Although he was also afraid of residual ankle pain, when he took the Percocet, he noticed that the pain of his current life situation would go away, too.

> The joke among medical professionals is that occasionally patients come in requesting Percocet for life pain. Most doctors say, "Too bad, it doesn't work." My point is that it *does* work. It actually works really well. Narcotics treat life pain for a short period of time very well. It treats all types of pain: existential pain, spiritual pain, physical pain, all pain, because they work on the brain where pain is processed. I started taking it for my life pain, essentially.

Bob Levy had what is called a paradoxical reaction to opioids: they did not make him sleepy. It almost made him feel as if he had consumed a lot of coffee, and he started to do better in school. Because his parents were doctors and many family friends were as well, he convinced them all to keep writing him prescriptions based on his ankle pain, surgery, recovery, and "flare ups." When he was worried about being in pain while he was taking the MCAT exams, he "took a bunch of Vicodin" for that, hoping he would do better on the tests. He was never sure what an effect that had, but he did get into medical school.

Because his ankle was still a problem, he decided to delay medical school for a year to rehabilitate it and learn to walk on it again. He moved home to New York and began working out and feeling good; he cut his pills down to once a week or so. Because he was still in physical pain, he could take them intermittently without suffering from any withdrawal symptoms. "Although it is hard to be your own doctor," he retrospectively diagnosed himself at this point in his life as someone who was abusing narcotics but wasn't addicted to them—yet. According to the Diagnostic and Statistical Manual of Mental Disorders, 5th ed., it would be considered "mild opioid use disorder." After getting back on his feet, Levy spent the rest of the year working at a ski resort in Aspen, Colorado, and described himself as being lonely and bored. He still had plenty of Vicodin and used them every couple of days. Once he began getting medical school interviews, he would take them before the interviews, again, to help with his anxiety. Then during the first year of medical school, he "almost never took them." The second year was harder because his fiancé was away at graduate school most evenings, so he began taking more. This pattern of using more, cutting back, and using more again went on throughout his four years of medical school. His wife never knew he was taking them—not at any point during their courtship, wedding, or early marriage.

When the time came to decide on a specialty, his choices were anesthesia or family medicine. He chose anesthesia and landed a prestigious residency in a large university hospital. He experienced withdrawal from opiates but didn't realize it and then used only intermittently the first year of residency. By the second year, he was finished with the other specialty rotations and settled into doing more anesthesia-related work. Levy soon began to feel bored about the choice he had made and realized that although he respected it and his colleagues very much, it didn't suit his desire to be interacting with patients. "At the same time, I am running out of pills. Most of my doctors, or suppliers, frankly, are in New York. I am not. I am far away from New York. I would go back to New York for vacations and hit these people up for more drugs and they would give them to me because I am so-and-so's son." It had now been five years since his ankle surgery. He started to get questions, and some stopped writing him prescriptions. He remembered, "I needed more and more, and my supply was dwindling, and I couldn't go back [to New York] as much."

One day it happens, I was basically out. Like most drug addicts, I was hypercareful about my supply, and I was down to my emergency supply. I went to work, and I went into withdrawal for the first time at the hospital, and that was really terrible. . . .

Sweating, shaking not so much, diarrhea, abdominal cramps, not looking healthy, having a runny nose, yawning, tearing up . . . full on withdrawal. . . .

Every addict has a way of dealing. I am doing what I can and managing as best I can. I know I wasn't [doing well] because my attending [physician] was kind of like, "What is going on? Get your shit together." I got nervous. I remember [for] the first time, thinking, "Well, fentanyl is a narcotic. It's right there and I know how to use it." At the time I thought of it as borrowing, but it was really stealing. I stole fentanyl for the first time.

Dr. Levy started using fentanyl by dividing it between himself and his patients. He doesn't defend his behavior at all, knowing that all of the medicine was intended for patients only. He knew he wanted to be done with using when he began his residency months before this moment and emphatically explained to me that it was "against every ethical and moral thing I stood for . . . and it still took me like fifteen months to come to the point where I was like, 'Okay, it's time.'"

Intravenous fentanyl is a "big jump" from opiate pain pills. Not long after Levy started doing this, his life began to fall apart. "The withdrawals are a million times worse. The cravings start, and they are really bad." His wife began noticing his strange behavior, his friends asked what was going on, and his attending anesthesiologist saw the signs. "I was the poster child: I was taking more bathroom breaks, I was volunteering for call, I was wearing long sleeves—I had to wear long sleeves because I had track marks at this point. I normally do not wear long sleeves and I was doing it all the time now at this point, and it wasn't because I was cold!" He had tried to quit many times, by tapering, substituting, and even tried to induce withdrawal by using naloxone. The anxiety around completely stopping was a big driver in his inability to seek help outside himself, but thankfully for Levy, anesthesiologists are often keenly aware of the signs of drug use among colleagues.

His attending physician knew exactly what she had to do, and she followed the well-established protocols in place for her to effectively handle this case. Levy had just finished a cardiac rotation, and one of his patients woke up in a lot of pain, despite charts that said he had been given plenty of narcotic pain relief. This is when she knew for sure that he was using. All the signs had been there, but this confirmed it. Bob had a great deal of respect for his supervising doctor, and she knew about things in his personal life that had been difficult for him that past year—his parents' divorce, his father remarrying, his mother moving to live closer to him, and then his aunt dying—so when she called him into her office that Saturday, he knew something was up. At first, he denied it. She remained completely silent. Then he broke into sobs. She told him it was okay, that she'd be driving him home, and then asked for his pager. At his house, she came in with him to be there when he told his wife what happened. Then she asked him to show them where in the house he had any other drugs hidden.

> For whatever reason, I was completely honest. I showed them where all of them were, and they threw away all of them. So, I had no access from the first time, which was the day that I broke my ankle. From March 15, 2001, until May 3, 2008, I was always within reach of a narcotic. And that was the first day that I was not. It was scary.
>
> At the same time, it was liberating. That withdrawal, although it was really bad, in my mind was not nearly as bad as the other ones because I was never thinking about how I was going to get more, what I was going to do, how I was going to hide it. I was like, "fuck it, it's out." I do remember distinctly thinking how I was never going to be happy again. I do remember that. The only thing that made me happy was drugs. . . . I just knew I was going to have to live without ever being happy again—which is not true.

Even though he surely has grumpy days, it is hard to imagine Bob Levy not being happy, in an overarching kind of way. He shared his recovery story with such enthusiasm, despite the many consequences and frustrations he endured as a result of his opioid addiction. A few days into his withdrawal, he went to an intake appointment with an addiction medicine doctor who decided against offering him buprenorphine but did recommend an intensive outpatient program, which Levy began attending. He also started going to AA meetings, got a sponsor, and dealt with the state medical board. After some time, they came back with the decision that he had to go to an inpatient program that specialized in treating doctors with addiction issues. He chose a twenty-eight-day, out-of-state program, but when he arrived, he learned it was actually ninety days. Although he was put on leave at the hospital, when he returned, he was terminated; this despite a pre-treatment plan to switch to family medicine. In the eyes of the hospital administrators, simply switching to family medicine didn't ameliorate his prior missteps, so they let him go. His wife, supportive as she was, decided around this time that she wanted to be closer to family in Minnesota and that she was moving there, hoping he would join her. He scrambled to find a residency in Minnesota, and despite the odds stacked against him so late in the year, he found one.

How addiction medicine came to be a specialty in his practice is a story that weaves together his own addiction, his treatment program, and his parents' vocations as psychiatrists. The program where he was accepted was in family medicine at North Memorial Hospital in Minneapolis. His own addiction treatment provider inspired him to study addiction medicine.

> When I first got intervened on, I initially thought that addicts are bad people.
>
> I'm sorry; I did think that. Through treatment, I thought, "Well, other addicts aren't bad people, but I'm a bad person." Part of Dr. Williams's approach was teaching us about the disease. He said, "You're not a bad person. I know you did some bad things, I'm not going to lie. But this is why. This is what is happening in your brain."
>
> I found that fascinating. My parents are both psychiatrists. I knew I didn't want to do psychiatry. I wanted to do something that was more medical, and this seemed like a great intersection. I was just utterly fascinated about it, and I started reading about it in treatment.

Months later, at the University of Minnesota's North Memorial Clinic, he found himself in the surprising position of being somewhat of an expert on addiction, even among his supervisors. Addiction was not taught in family medicine training, or in any kind of medical school training, actually. He realized that no one knew the first thing about addiction. In exchanges he described like this, he tried to make them understand.

> They would say, "This guy is an alcoholic. He's in bad pain, we should just give him Percocet."

"That's a bad idea."

"Why?"

"What do you mean, why?"

"He's addicted to alcohol, he's not going to get addicted to Percocet."

"That's not how it goes!"

Dr. Levy, then a second-year resident, began printing articles and showing them to the attending physicians, who were genuinely open to learning about addiction. Scant medical school training about the science of addiction existed, even as recently as 2009, and he found himself regularly teaching his superiors and colleagues about it.

And so his passion for addiction treatment in primary care settings began. "Addiction treatment belongs in primary care. Not all of it, there is a time and a place for an addiction specialist, but like diabetes, the vast majority of addiction treatment, I feel, should occur in primary care settings." Through his growing network of healthcare professionals in recovery, he was encouraged to approach Hazelden about the possibility of creating a fellowship position in addiction medicine for him, where he could work and be mentored. They agreed, so his residency was split between the University of Minnesota and Hazelden.

The consequences of his addiction followed him through rigorous state medical licensing requirements, and so for three and a half years into his time in Minnesota, he had to call in every day to find out if it was his day for a random urine drug screen. The state also required quarterly reports from his work supervisors and his AA sponsor. In addition to that, he recounted, "I needed to have meeting attendance, I had to see a psychiatrist, I had to do aftercare again. . . . I had been sober for two years. They suddenly mandated that I had to do another aftercare program. . . . But I was still at the stage where I was like, okay, whatever." He had to attend twenty-five two-hour meetings related to addiction and recovery with others in recovery and, smiling, recalled, "It was great, actually." Although he complied with every requirement the state mandated—he was at risk of losing his medical license if he didn't—he felt that recovery and all things associated with it were so good that it was easy to comply. And yet Dr. Levy also acknowledged that while he had certain personal strengths growing up, "humility was not one of them." Then he continued, humbly, "I'm not sure you could call humility one of my strengths now, but I certainly have a lot more of it than I did. I wouldn't call it one of my weaknesses anymore." When he was a patient himself at Hazelden, he realized that he did not have all the answers about his addiction and that he needed to learn to listen to those with more experience if he was going to stay sober. He abided this common AA practice then and continues to believe that "when I start to take control of my disease is when I start to run into trouble."

Another aspect of recovery for Dr. Levy has been being open about his struggle with addiction, both personally and professionally. Now as an attending physician himself, he is completely transparent about his own past struggles. "I tell them in orientation about my own story as a part of wellness. I say, 'Look, there are fourteen people in this room between the staff and the residents. Statistically, two of us are going to develop a problem with substance use disorder. Fortunately for you guys, I have already taken one of the spots." He always tells them that if something comes up, he is there for whoever needs him, and over the years, some have come forward for help.

The continued level of stigma around addiction among healthcare professionals can only be reduced by positive, open interactions with people in recovery and by better training in substance use disorders and treatments. Levy is working on that with every group of residents he teaches. "Every year we graduate ten family medicine doctors and none of them . . . are going to blindly prescribe benzos or narcotics to anyone with an opioid use disorder. They will at least have a conversation about risks and benefits and monitor them with drug screening." In most family medicine settings, screening for drug use via questionnaire or conversation is not standard practice, and he believes this is due to the lack of education physicians received about addiction in medical school. "Part of the reason doctors don't screen for addiction is because you will never convince a physician to screen for something . . . that they have no idea how to treat. They would just prefer to not ask the question. No one wants to feel like an idiot." Screening tools have been developed, such as SBIRT (screening, brief intervention, and referral to treatment), and have proved successful in studies for some drugs and in some healthcare settings, but Levy would like to see these kinds of simple screenings thoroughly and consistently integrated into primary care.[25]

Once they are screened, though, the doctor also has to know what to do if an issue is discovered. What are the next steps? Where do they refer patients? Even knowing all he does and working in the "Land of 10,000 Rehabs," as Minnesota is jokingly referred to in some circles, he is often frustrated by the lack of immediate treatment options once a patient has agreed to get help. Even as a primary care physician, he can't pull strings to get a patient into treatment quickly, and this troubles him immensely.

> Right now—when you are ready—you need to go directly to treatment. . . . Even [waiting] a day is too much. Sometimes even twelve hours is too much. . . . I want to see a primary care doctor that says, "This guy needs help right now," like you would if someone was having a heart attack. You would get them a bed at the hospital immediately. You are not going to wait two days on a heart attack.

Comparing serious substance use disorder with a heart attack or diabetes comes naturally to Dr. Levy, and all the other physicians who see addiction as a medical condition. Another way to reduce stigma is to keep making these kinds of comparisons. Not long ago, cancer was considered a socially unspeakable diagnosis, referred to as "the C word."[26] Integrating basic substance use disorder screening into primary-care interactions would destigmatize it considerably, not to mention reduce the number of emergency room visits related to it. In Levy's perfect world, primary care doctors would understand substance use disorder as well as they understand heart disease; they would know when a patient needs to be referred to an addiction specialist, just like they would refer one to a cardiologist. In his family medicine practice, Levy sees primarily opioid-dependent patients and lets his residents see the patients with the most common substance use disorder, alcoholism.

As for the relationship between his personal experience and his skills as an addiction medicine specialist, he thinks it may be easier for him, but it surely isn't necessary in order to be a good, understanding physician. Colleagues who work in emergency medicine think he is "crazy" for working in addiction medicine, but Levy explained to them that he sees patients in recovery, who are being treated effectively for their addiction, not the people who tend to show up in the ER in crisis, overdose, or worse. "They come to see us, they know that they have a problem, and they are there to work with us to get better. They are not the patients in the ER screaming for meds. They are not the pain patients that every doctor hates to see." And, as if speaking directly to his physician colleagues, he concluded the interview with this:

> That pain patient that you hate to see, you hate to see because he or she has an addiction problem. If you confront it, then you have one painful visit and you can help them get over it. . . . Just get it over with, confront them, or discuss it with them. . . . That is the crux of recovery in a lot of ways. . . . Once it is out in the open, they can yell at you and scream at you. It can be a tough visit. I do this a lot, and my heart rate still goes up when I go into the room. Then we get to move on.

Andrew Tuttle, PhD, MD

A few years ago, I had the opportunity to go to Switzerland to meet two doctors, Andy Tuttle, a psychiatrist who is the brother of a family friend in St. Paul, and Thilo Beck, the director of an addiction medicine clinic in Zurich, whom Andy had arranged for us to meet during my short stay. Arud Center for Addiction Medicine is a comprehensive outpatient clinic located in a modern, colorful, and plant-filled office space. Dr. Beck gave us a tour and sat for an interview. I had no idea then what an impact that hour would make on me. Meeting Thilo Beck and visiting his clinic has forever changed my perspective about what is possible when it comes to solving substance use disorders in the United States. By not offering adequate medical treatment and consistent, human rights–oriented access to support services, not only have we created the problem in the first place, we have continued to perpetuate and feed it. Even just looking at the revolving door of drug and alcohol treatment, we are simply not applying the knowledge and science we have accumulated in an effective, broad manner. Yes, Switzerland is wealthy and small, but it also had a terrible heroin epidemic in the early 1990s, one that it completely resolved in a matter of years.[27] Today in Switzerland, heroin is a drug of the past, once used by "old people," as the youth there tend to view it. The information and pragmatism he offered were both overwhelming and refreshing to behold. One of the most powerful insights Dr. Beck shared with me that morning in Zurich was this:

> Saying opioid addiction is a chronic disease may be true, but I think it is a chronic disease because the addicted people were not entrenched in it by their own fault. That disease is a result of the political and societal conditions we have had. The heroin addicts were forced into this marginalized lifestyle. They were made chronic. They were impaired not by the action of the substance of heroin, but of the side effects of illegal lifestyle and these horrible years they went through.[28]

Andy Tuttle and I had decided earlier that the afternoon would be a good time to record his interview, once we were back in his town, a short train ride from Zurich. Dr. Tuttle, in a turtleneck and jeans, tucked his long legs under him on the low-slung modern couch, and the family cat soon found a spot nearby to keep an eye on us. Tuttle's voice was consistently on the quiet side, so I used a stack of books to get the microphone closer to him.

My head was still kind of spinning after listening to Dr. Beck share how the Swiss model for addiction medicine and treatment developed, and how they treat people with substance abuse issues so completely differently than we do in the United States. I wondered if the reason for their divergent and highly successful approach was due to a combination of factors: their horrible heroin crisis of the 1990s, their democratic, legislative process whereby *every law* is voted on by the citizens, and their much more rational, culturally supported attitude about science and its ability to solve problems. When I asked Dr. Beck about how much stigma still exists regarding drug users, he seemed to believe there was still stigma in Switzerland. But from my vantage point, it almost didn't matter if stigma was still around because of what an incredibly effective job the Swiss did of nearly eradicating opioid addiction and truly treating substance use disorder for what it is—a manageable medical diagnosis.

Dr. Tuttle understood both societies quite well, and in this way, his life story became a bridge between Minnesota and Switzerland, between the Minnesota Model and the Four Pillars model of Swiss drug treatment: prevention, therapy, harm reduction, and law enforcement.[29]

Tuttle has been a psychiatrist in Baden, Switzerland, since the 1990s. He and his wife opened their home to me, a near total stranger, and gave me not only a lovely place to stay, but access to interviews and personal stories that turned out to be poignantly relevant to my project.

Born in Minneapolis in 1952, Andy Tuttle spent the first years of his childhood with well-educated, loving parents who also happened to have dramatic and bitter verbal battles with each other. His father worked at Gedney Pickles, where he would become CEO, and his mother was an English literature major in college, who later worked as a librarian in research laboratories and universities. Andy described himself as a difficult child and particularly remembered the way he was met with disapproval from adults. The school called his parents about his behavior constantly. He was the one who other children knew would do whatever they dared him to, and then they would go tell on him. "I was a troublemaker. I got into fights, and I was just hyperactive. I was all over the place." He was also smart and curious. Chuckling now, he remembered that when he was just six years old, he took his father's bicycle completely apart with tools he found in the garage. "Retrospectively, I most certainly had ADHD."[30]

By age ten, Andy's mother and father were divorced. Andy, his mother, and new stepfather traveled on a steamship to Switzerland where his stepfather had work with the Swiss Institute of Technology as a physicist for what would later become the Paul Scherrer Institute. Fighting between his mother and her new husband was again commonplace and had also become physical. "Only now with a certain temporal distance and knowing what I know about psychology and dealing with life myself, I know that she was a very, very emotionally difficult person, one that could get somebody to fight with her." At that point, though, he admitted she was *the* central person in his childhood, the only consistent relationship he had, so he managed their violent relationship as best he could.

Andy found Switzerland to be a great adventure, and he suddenly had room enough and challenges enough to keep his undiagnosed ADHD abated. They lived in a tiny farming village where he attended a small, multigrade schoolhouse with a teacher who had a very firm but gentle kind of authority. "Everybody just naturally did what he wanted," he explained, still a bit in awe of the man. Andy picked up

Swiss German easily and excelled at school, despite his perennial issue with unfinished homework assignments. He eventually made it into the more rigorous high school option and chose the natural sciences division because he excelled in those subjects.

The summer he was sixteen, Andy went back to Minneapolis to visit his father, who had by that time remarried and had two more sons. Andy had been stressed by his home life in Switzerland, so he asked to stay and live with his father, who was pleased and happy to have him. His father enrolled him in a private college preparatory school that year, one where most of the students had known each other for years already; he felt isolated and alienated. He didn't make friends easily, and none of the adults in his life ever realized he might be having a hard time adjusting to a new place because he spoke English like a local and excelled at school.

One day he just ran away. He took a bus to Chicago O'Hare and "presented a sob story to the Swiss people there, that I had been stranded in America." They confirmed he had parents there and put him on a plane home. He felt terrible about not talking to his father first but took it as his own personal failure and nothing his father had caused. Back in Switzerland, living again with his mom and stepfather, he remembered that he dove right into the "psychedelic hippie stuff" but never overdid it.

Andy moved out of his mother's house when he was nineteen. Although he now had three half sisters in Switzerland and three half brothers in Minnesota, he always felt like a single kid. "I knew how to be alone." He finished school, and then took a year off to work and travel. He bought a 1951 BMW motorcycle and toured Europe, the United States, and Central America. His mother died of breast cancer when he was twenty-three, and his stepfather died the year he finished medical school, in 1980. He married Susan Laube in 1982, had two sons, and eventually opened a private practice in Switzerland after having worked in a psychiatric hospital for several years.

When I asked Andy about how his practice has changed over the past three decades, and if his attitude toward people with addiction had changed over the years, he didn't give me the answer I expected. I imagined he would confirm what Thilo Beck had said earlier in the day, that heroin users have nearly disappeared in Switzerland, that they have aged out, and that he has fewer of them in his practice. He did say these things later, but just before that academic explanation, he got a little more pensive. "It's been a long road. It has a lot to do with my personal experience, too, a lot of personal stuff and realizing how vulnerable I am. [Addiction] is not something that is just a bad life choice . . . this is something that can happen to you . . . [it] took me completely by surprise." Shortly before he opened his own private practice, an anesthesiologist friend who had just received a permit to order opioid treatment pharmaceuticals suggested that the two of them "see what this whole thing is about, this flash." I asked him to clarify. "The flash, the rush, when you inject an opiate." Their first dose was too strong, and Andy remembered feeling woozy and too sleepy. The next time he tried it, he used a much smaller amount.

Just as Bob Levy had described to me, the effect of the drug was overwhelmingly positive. "That was, 'Oh my God.' All my troubles with attention deficit disorder, my problems with concentration, my problems with the strenuousness, with keeping up a conversation with anybody, and staying focused on the subject and not drifting away mentally, and my ability to read and retain stuff was just better." He started using it twice a week because it was helpful, but soon he began to feel discouraged because of the cravings in between. He got addicted. "This was a very, very profoundly humiliating experience." He elaborated, "I never thought that could happen to me. It never did with any other substance. I can smoke a joint tomorrow and then not think about it for a year. I like a glass of wine, but I don't crave it. I could easily go days or weeks without it. I had cocaine, I didn't like the effect because it made me all tight and nervous and crabby."

Andy's struggle with morphine lasted on and off for about ten years. "I detoxed three or four times. . . . I'm clean [now] but I'd still call myself an addict. I have vast amounts of oral morphine in my practice because I have to distribute it. [But] I never ever, ever keep injectable morphine in my practice. I know that it's too tempting." The humiliation was realizing that he was not in control of his use of the substance. He gained a much deeper understanding of what his patients go through as a result of his own "brush with morphine," as he called it. He understands deeply how a person can be thinking rationally and then do something completely contrary. "I am knowing as I'm doing it that I don't want to do it, but I'm doing it anyways. Here it is. 'Oh my God, that feels good. Why did I do that? What an asshole, now I did it again.'" He shared another aspect of it:

The other part is like somebody else is holding the steering wheel and driving you. It's a profound thing and I think it's kind of unique for the opiates. They have such an intricate, specific way of inter-acting with the receptors in your brain. They quickly, after a rela-tively short time, can change the way that your brain is function-ing and the way of steering your thoughts and your behavior.

He admitted that while he was a compassionate and thoughtful doctor before this, he understood so much more about addiction during and after his own struggles. Pinching his thumb and index finger together, with just a slight space of light between them, he said, "I never feel, ever, even this much superiority over my patients. I know why they lie. I know how that works. I know how much they hate themselves for lying. The whole shame thing and everything is just mind-blowing."

Emily Brunner Youseff, MD

Before she left for her first year of college, Emily Brunner's grand-mother offered her $1,000 if she could get through college without drinking alcohol. She decided it wasn't worth it and laughed as she re-layed this story about her family history of alcoholism. Brunner grew up in Ridgefield, Connecticut, the daughter of a physicist and a choir teacher, with alcoholism and heavy alcohol use on both sides of her family. Her paternal grandfather was the person most remembered for this, and she knew from an early age it was a difficult subject for her mom. Her parents never drank, and yet she learned at an early age how to drink alcohol adults left around at parties. The oldest of four siblings, Emily described herself as an "uber nerd" with just a few debate team friends in high school. During her junior year, the team went to a meet at MIT. Trusted by the chaperones and left to their own in the dorms, they quickly "developed a plan to infiltrate an MIT frat party." There, she got drunk and kissed a boy for the first time and remembered, "I loved being drunk."[31] Although this happened only a few times in high school (because she got in a lot of trouble), from the very beginning of her drinking years Brunner admitted that she drank to black out.

She ended up going to MIT for college, as her father had, and ini-tially intended to become an engineer "because not many women go into engineering." She realized by her junior year that she didn't like it and switched to premed. She drank heavily throughout college. When asked if she ever thought it was a problem, or if she wanted to drink less, she describes a common aspect of addiction: justification and denial.

> I certainly had a lot of negative experiences related to it, and I stopped drinking for thirty days once just to prove that I didn't have a problem. The thing that sort of perpetuated me thinking it was okay was that I continued to be able to pull it out for tests. I had a pretty high GPA, and it wasn't interfering with that aspect of things, and that made it feel okay. . . . I definitely gravitated toward people who drank heavily, and I blacked out a lot, but I liked it. I really liked it. . . . It's amazing how potently biological that part was.

When she made the decision to apply to medical schools, she said she was able to "sort of pull it together and stop for a while in that period." Although she had planned to specialize in cardiology or some other specialty, once she was on rotations as a resident, she discovered she liked family medicine the most. "I felt it was a field where I could actually do the kind of medicine I pictured doctors doing when I was little and could answer questions for my family members. I really liked the variety of it."

During medical school rotations in 2006, Brunner discovered a large tumor in her abdomen that had to be removed immediately. Before surgery, she consented to having her reproductive organs removed, if necessary. She was living with her future husband, but until the tumor scare, she had not particularly wanted to have a family. This health issue changed her mind and brought a desire to have children to the forefront. Although the tumor turned out to be benign, the surgeon did have to take out one ovary and one fallopian tube. While she was recovering in the hospital she remembered that the first doctor she talked to gave her a prescription for Ativan and said, "Take as much as you want." She took a lot. "I loved it. It was sort of pill alcohol." She used Ativan intermittently for the next three years.

In 2007, she and her boyfriend married before she began her residency. They thought they would try to get pregnant at some point during her residency, assuming it would take longer due to her prior surgery. It didn't. She discovered she was pregnant right when she began the internship. It was a really challenging experience, both physically and with her fellow residents. "I really tried to not do anything differently than the other residents because they were sort of irritated with me; if I was out they would have to do more work. In fact, one of them, [during] the first days of our residency tried to have us make a pact that none of us would get pregnant during the intern year, and I said, 'I'm not making that pact.' It was uncomfortable." Brunner remembered feeling sad and isolated during this time in her life. She was far away from medical school friends and her family in Connecticut; she was newly married and working too hard. After twenty-one days in a row without a day off, she started having contractions at only twenty weeks pregnant. She was put on bed rest and sank into a depression.

She wasn't drinking or using pills when she was pregnant but remembered getting out a bottle of Ativan and counting the pills. Contemplating that behavior now, she says, "That was a little weird." She went full term but had "a scary delivery" in March 2008. While recuperating from the birth, she was prescribed a "huge supply of oxycodone," her first exposure to opioids. After that bottle ran out, she called and had it refilled. "At that point I had never heard anyone say addiction was an illness. I thought the way I drank was probably not right, but I really didn't know what was wrong with me. I was trying all kinds of antidepressants, I had postpartum depression, and it was really just an awful period of time." She struggled with returning to her medical residency. As so many new mothers with careers admit, she felt trapped. "I loved my daughter so much. I had never experienced anything like that—loving someone so much—and when I had to go back to work it really broke my heart." She spoke with the residency director and he told her, "Well, either come back or don't come back, but there's no way we can work out any kind of schedule." She learned that this was not true, but took his response as a sign that he wasn't willing to work something out with her.

After she went back to work, her prescription had run out, so she began using alcohol more frequently. She also started to see a "secret residency doctor" to help her with the mental health issues that had arisen during her pregnancy and postpartum. This doctor prescribed her a lot of Ativan, and she combined that with alcohol. Before long, she began having back pain that, at first, she believed was legitimate. Her use cascaded quickly into serious addiction-related behaviors. "I remember thinking, I know medicine, and no one can tell me I *don't* have back pain, and so I was doing physical therapy but also using oxycodone. At first it was prescribed, and then I was just picking it up and taking it and just crossing all kinds of—I mean, I descended into a person I didn't recognize quite quickly." She recalled this as "a terrible period of time in her life," the details unnecessary, except to share that she had become a person she no longer recognized. She went into treatment in 2009.

Dr. Brunner considered herself very lucky to have been evaluated by a doctor she still believes was "probably the best addiction medicine doctor I've ever seen practice." In recovery himself, Dr. Patrick Gibbons was beloved by people from all sectors of his life and career— his colleagues, his patients, and many who worked in mental health, addiction medicine, and recovery. Brunner remembered hating him at first because he held her to such a high standard, but "he was an amazing, wonderful mentor and doctor."[32] He referred her to Talbott, a specialized addiction treatment center designed for the professional needs of doctors and pilots in Atlanta, Georgia, named after its founder, Dr. G. Douglas Talbott. The "special needs" of these professionals may be related to professional standards, ethics violations, and more, but in her colleague Bob Levy's experience, it ultimately comes down to the humiliating and intense fear of losing their licenses, whether to fly or practice medicine—they would rather die.

In Dr. Brunner's experience, her time at Talbott also taught her about addiction in ways her medical training never had. Remembering this, she exclaimed, "What the hell, this is a disease? Why didn't someone tell me? I had learned the side effects of liver disease from alcohol, but not that there was any hope for people stopping, or that there are medications to treat alcohol [use]. . . . And I went to med school during the period where it was like, if you have pain, we have to treat it. Pain is a vital sign. You can't get addicted to opiates if you have real pain."

She now knows how wrong that information was and has her own experiences to back it up. After completing treatment, Brunner had to repeat her second year of residency in family medicine, and then decided to pursue addiction medicine as a specialty. She abided by every requirement to fulfill her residency as well as followed all the rules related to the chemical dependency monitoring program for three years. Once she completed that, she moved with her family to Minnesota to work at Hazelden.

Roughly two years prior to her taking the job there, Hazelden had slowly begun to integrate limited medications for some clients with opioid use disorder, particularly Vivitrol, and tapered Suboxone use.[33] The use of Suboxone was controversial not only at Hazelden, but also among physicians in recovery from addiction. This did not sit well with her. After working with opioid-dependent young adults at Hazelden, Brunner came to the conclusion that abstinence-only, Twelve Step treatment for chronic opiate users, even under twenty-six, is inadequate. "It's hard to watch all the misinformation about Suboxone go through the world. It is a medication that reduces the risk of relapse and death by 50 to 75 percent and is hugely effective, and we do not employ it with the vast majority of patients. They're dying. I'm tired of watching; it breaks my heart."

The stigma against using medications for opioid use disorder remains among the most frustrating aspects of her job to this day. "There's still certainly a lot of pejorative stigma surrounding Suboxone, language around not being 'clean' if you're on it, which I think kills people. If I'm prescribing someone a medication they are taking as prescribed, then they are abstinent. I hate when people tell them that they're not." Although she has found great support in Twelve Step programs for herself, and will suggest them when appropriate, the life-saving and life-sustaining properties that evidence-based medications offer patients are imperative to curbing the epidemic. "I think that it's pretty scientifically established how you treat opiate use disorder. I don't see that being implemented the way that it needs to be."

Sober since 2009, Emily Brunner doesn't take her recovery for granted, nor her weaknesses, nor the hard lessons learned in her own life. Being forthcoming with her own substance use issues has paid off, especially with her personal physicians. "When I go to the doctor, sometimes I say, 'I've been sober for seven and a half years.' I tell it to them the first time I go, but there are a lot of people in sobriety who don't. Doctors can be real idiots about treating it. I went to the ER six months ago for an ear infection, and they offered me morphine. They didn't ask me. And I was able to [tell them] but, you know, there are probably days where that could have ruined my life." She applies her personal experience to her work with patients at St. Joseph's, where she has been since 2016, working more directly with a wider variety of people in an outpatient addiction medicine setting. The majority of her patients are on Suboxone, and she knows that one or two of them are in active relapse every day. "A lot of what I do is try to check for mental health, talk to them in a way that's nonjudgmental, exhibits caring, and I get urine drug screens from everyone I see, regardless of how long they've been sober, because you just never know."

What frustrates Dr. Brunner the most is that care delivery and other related systems aren't coordinated. "We're not well networked between the medical field, the healthcare field, even the research field, the CD [chemical dependency] world, and the legal world. It's all split up, and that kills people, and I hate that because it's actually not that complicated to treat." She cited a lack of resources as a problem, noting a lack of Suboxone providers, sober housing, and other services, even in a state well known for having more recovery resources than most. Her comment that addiction is "not that complicated to treat" reveals the dissonance between the medical and scientific understanding of addiction and the morality-based stigma, shame, and personal responsibility model that has kept a tight rein on how addiction has been treated. Dr. Brunner is active in addiction medicine organizations and works to promote the increased use of medications for opioid dependence, locally and nationally. She is keenly aware of the challenges ahead and sees increasing problems with drugs besides opioids: benzodiazepines and methamphetamine are on the rise. She remains very committed to the work of addiction medicine. "I really love what I do. I feel really blessed and proud and happy, and it's kind of not where I ever thought I would be. I had no plans to move to Minnesota, be an addiction medicine doctor, and have a lovely family; like objectively, that was not the plan. It's so much better than I would have guessed."

Marv Seppala, MD

If one person's story could embody both the benefits of a Twelve Step–based recovery and the overwhelming need for evidence-based addiction medicine treatments during the opioid epidemic, it is Marv Seppala's life and work. As a person in long-term recovery and a psychiatrist who specializes in addiction medicine, Seppala's career combined two fields that had long been at opposite ends of treatment solutions for addiction. Psychiatry was not practiced in early addiction treatment centers—in fact, the treatment of alcoholics by psychiatrists and physicians was exactly what the architects of the Minnesota

Model were trying to escape: the sanatoriums and inebriate asylums that as late as 1950 still housed alcoholics and the mentally ill together. Derided and described as "snake pits," midcentury mental health reformers in Minnesota didn't know what exactly to do with the "inebs," as they were called colloquially. Dan Anderson, one of these reformers, and among the founders of the Minnesota Model, put their predicament bluntly when he said, "We agreed that alcoholism was an illness—at least we were going to make believe it was until somebody explained it better."[34]

Marv Seppala's life and career would come to span both the success of the new model as well as its failures. He made it his life's work to integrate them, despite being taken to task by the stalwarts of Twelve Step abstinence as well as the science-led experts of the medical model. Seppala is a gifted storyteller, and despite the painful content, we laughed many times with an ease that surprised me since we had never met before. His quick smile, humble demeanor, and laid-back personality nearly made me forget I was finally interviewing the chief medical officer of the Hazelden Betty Ford Foundation.

Marv Seppala was born in Seattle in 1956, the first of five siblings, to his Finnish-born mother and Finnish Minnesotan father. The Seppalas had moved every four years—Seattle, San Jose, and then to Eden Prairie, Minnesota, a suburb of Minneapolis, when Marv was eight. When he was twelve, they settled in Stewartville, Minnesota, a town thirteen miles south of Rochester, home to the famed Mayo Clinic. Although he described his mother as a housewife, she had also been a famous Finnish cross-country ski champion. His dad was a chemical engineer for the shiny, new IBM plant in Rochester, located on a sprawling four-hundred-acre campus. A self-conscious, anxious kid, Marv recalled that the multiple moves took a bit of a toll on him. But ever the optimist, as I quickly noticed, he said that after living in big cities, it was easier to make friends in a town with one school and one class of kids in his grade.

In 1970, the town of Stewartville had a population of around 2,800 and was surrounded by fields and forests, especially along the north branch of Root River. Marv had a lot of stories to tell about early escapades with friends, floating on river ice chunks, breaking into the gun club to warm up, sneaking alcohol, and shooting at small things with a .22 caliber. In other words, an idyllic Midwestern childhood. Kids—well, boys more likely—were free to roam.

His hugely entertaining stories were braided with his first experiences with alcohol. The summer between sixth and seventh grade,
Marv was hanging out with a few friends at a farm. They snuck some
whiskey out of the kitchen and went to the barn. "I remember I just
could hardly understand why anyone would swallow this stuff. It
tasted so bad. It burnt my throat—and then all of a sudden—feeling
like I belonged. Like I was part of these other two guys who had grown
up together and I no longer had these worries or fears about that or
anything else, really. It was like I was suddenly part of the world or
something." He recalled feeling as if his whole life changed, and he
knew he would do it again. He didn't drink again until the next summer and, after that, more frequently. "It was really remarkable. . . . It
felt like I was part of something for the first time, and that is a strange
thing to describe."[35]

Athletics and academics were valued in his family, and Marv especially looked up to the athletes at his school. Since junior high and
high school students were in the same building, by seventh grade, he
had ample opportunities to hang out with athletes and older kids. One
of those was the older brother of a friend, both an athlete and a good
student. When he returned from his first year at the University of
Minnesota, he told his younger brother and Marv about smoking pot,
"its importance and how fun it was," and although Marv remembered
thinking, "I will never do that," within a week, he had tried it and liked
it. As a clinician looking back on his life, he had a very interesting perspective of peer pressure, one that seemed almost the exact opposite
of the typical narrative about the evils of peer pressure.

> I have certainly read about peer pressure and thought about [it]
> in regard to its influence on people. When I look back on my own
> life in regard to substance use, I was always pushing the envelope
> and seeking more substance use, and I needed to find people
> who were doing the same, so that I wouldn't stick out. Once I got
> going, I didn't want people to know how often I was using, how
> much I was using, all of the different drugs I was using. . . . I had
> to hang out with people who were doing the same so I wouldn't
> feel as bad.

The guilt he had about using drugs was easier to deal with if he hung
around kids who were doing the same—"so I wouldn't feel as bad." That

sounded right, and seemed more to do with feeling part of something than simply feeling pressured to try something.

Marv's use of alcohol and then other assorted drugs escalated beginning in eighth grade, but it wouldn't be until his senior year that his use spiraled out of his ability to control it. He managed to keep it from his parents by staying out late, telling them he was at one sports practice or another, but he didn't skip school—most of the time—though curfew breaking was a regular event. Despite being able to uphold day-to-day responsibilities, things became more complicated as he got older. In the span of four months, he was in six different car accidents as a passenger while driving with his friends. Parties usually involved a pile of sweet corn, a keg of beer, and other drugs, often spread out at farms outside town, on winding gravel roads. To my surprise, he remembered that only a couple of the accidents involved impaired driving. Marv was so shaken by these wrecks that for a while he refused to get in cars with his friends.

During Christmas break of his senior year, Marv had access to a lot of speed—in pill form, not joy rides. He proceeded to use it consistently for two weeks over the break. He had never used speed so frequently. The day before school started, he ran out. He didn't know about amphetamine withdrawal, but that was what happened in school that Monday. "I had no energy, I actually pretty much passed out in my precalculus class with my favorite teacher. I'm on my desk and I am just asleep, and I hear a yardstick slam on the desk and I just kind of look up momentarily, and I just went right back out." The school nurse called his family doctor who sent him to St. Mary's Hospital on the Mayo campus. No one asked him about drug use, and he didn't offer any information. They thought he had encephalitis or meningitis, so he had to have a spinal tap. The spinal tap leaked, and so he suffered with an intermittent headache for another week, on top of the amphetamine withdrawals he was still having. "They couldn't figure it out. Now I'm fine, except for the headache, which they caused!"

Marv laughed at the absurdity of this tale—no one had asked about or tested for drug use—because during the week he recuperated at home, he had a friend pick him up every day to get high while his mom was gone. He would always return home before she did. After a week or so of this, he told her that his headaches were gone and then told his school he was still home sick. His parents were beginning to catch on; eventually they found a pipe and papers in his car.

They still didn't press him, the consequences were minimal, and so his use continued.

Marv went back to school at some point, but shame caught up with him anyway. The day before a physics test, a class he really liked, his teacher asked him to solve a problem on the board to show the rest of the class. "I'm up there writing them out . . . they were easy to do because I had done my homework the night before. . . . I am all prepared!" That night, he went out and, as he described it, "got wasted smoking pot." In class the next day, the only thing he wrote on his test was his name. "I cannot remember how to do the problems that I was up at the board doing the day before. . . . I couldn't even answer one question. I walked out of the class and I walked out of school and I was so ashamed. . . . I just decided I wasn't going back. I didn't think it through that way, what I thought was 'I'm going to go get high and I am not going back.'" In spite of his drug use and missing school, Marv's grades had not suffered much, but this humiliation was more than he could process. He didn't go back to school. He moved a few doors down from his parents for a little while, but since he didn't have any money, he returned home, still determined to not finish high school. This was when his parents realized that Marv was in trouble. He was out using drugs and drinking "dawn to dusk," and said of that time, "I can't stand myself."

Of his emotional state and his lack of understanding about addiction, Marv explained what might on the surface seem naïve, but was incredibly heart-wrenching. His demeanor while sharing this seemed to channel the younger man he was then.

> I don't know that it is the drugs and alcohol. In fact, I think that is the only relief I get. I really don't think that [drug use] is the problem. I [do] think there is a big problem. I can't understand why I keep doing these things that I am so ashamed of—you know, stealing and lying. I've quit school, which I loved. I've been kicked out of sports by this point, which I really loved. And I don't know how to change any of this. . . . I'm not really even able to have plans, I couldn't figure out how to do it. I didn't know. I didn't have a clue and I couldn't tell anybody. I didn't want anyone to know how awful I felt.

Very early one morning, after a late night out partying, Marv was shaken awake by his mother and their family doctor, Dr. Riser. All Marv remembered him saying was, "Yeah, he's on something." He fell back to sleep and then was woken up again at six. But this time the local minister was in his bedroom, and his mother told Marv to get up because they were going to the hospital. He remembered that it didn't even occur to him then that this was unusual, so he just complied. They headed toward Rochester, which made sense since that was where they went for healthcare, but then they didn't stop. They kept driving and pulled into the IBM campus where Marv's dad was waiting. They got on the highway and headed toward Minneapolis. Marv learned later that their minister was poised in the back seat, just in case he decided to jump out of the car. He remembered feeling quite scared when they passed the Twin Cities and kept driving—since he already felt like he was going crazy, the idea crossed his mind that they might be taking him to some kind of "sanitarium in the North Woods." He assumed that was what happened to people like him.

As they drove onto a long driveway, Marv noticed a sign and then thought to himself, "What the hell is a Hazelden?" The first thing they did was introduce him to a counselor, who took him to an office to chat alone. The man was pleasant and likable. This stranger was the first person he had ever met who knew what was going on with him, who almost seemed to know him before actually knowing him. "It was just uncanny to me. I am shocked by this." Of course, the counselor knew addiction, but Marv didn't, so he was amazed. "I am just wondering who told him this, because I never tell my parents any of this, they couldn't have told him. . . . But he knows me somehow." Marv shared a few things with the counselor that he'd never said to anyone, and he then started to realize that in the counselor's mind, "I am clearly an addict." They wrapped up and went to meet with his parents. The plan was for Marv to stay for four weeks, and he just had to sign some papers first. Despite his hangover, inner turmoil, and despair, he did not submit willingly. He thought, "I do not want to stop getting high. I certainly don't want to stay here. I have never even heard of this [place]. And it's a threat, in a way." He refused to sign the papers. His father provided a bluff: he told Marv that if he didn't stay, they would get a judge to force treatment on him, to have the court commit him (though now he wondered aloud with me if that was even possible in the 1970s). The threat worked. He was very scared of any legal situation regarding his drug use, so he complied.

This was 1974. Marv was seventeen. As it turned out, he was the first teenager treated at Hazelden for chemical dependency—the new term of the time. Although Hazelden, established in 1949, had recently built more modern facilities, the original building, known as the Old Lodge, was still in use as a unit. Marv later learned that in the 1970s this was the unit reserved for people who had multiple issues and "more hardcore addictions." Although it is hard to imagine today, in the 1960s and 1970s, alcohol and drug use were treated separately and as distinctly different issues.[36] Marv's placement in the lodge fit with that history and yet also revealed that even though he was a teenager, Hazelden was willing to try treating him for polydrug use. He remembered that he was the youngest there by a long shot.

Marv spent the first two weeks of his four-week stay arguing that he didn't belong at Hazelden at all. He interrupted his narrative to tell me that he still has *The Big Book* from this time. He laughed as he told me about the cryptic little notes he had written in the margins about why he didn't belong there and why he wasn't an alcoholic. He even used the daily worksheets they had clients fill out, called a "significant events sheet," to explain in detail why he didn't belong there. Every morning, over the intercom system, someone would direct him to report to his counselor's office. His counselor would point out that Marv's arguments were wrong, not in a bullying way, but he just wanted to "talk it through." Marv didn't listen to the counselor.

But he listened in group. Looking back at his younger self, he can now solidly affirm the benefit of group therapy for addiction.

> In the midst of this resistance on my part that I might be an addict, that I can't even see, I can absolutely see it in everyone else in the group. I mean, they are describing it. Even if they believe it or not, I can see it. I mean, they have given all of these examples, you know? They've described their life and *they* should be here because of what they have been doing. And they're a lot older, but they have lost their jobs, they have lost families, and all of these things. And I can see it in them. And then, it finally starts to dawn on me that all of these examples that I am using about them are the same examples in my life.

Once he started to see his own behaviors, he realized that he had been accepted by his peers there all along, that they understood him and knew what he was going through. "And they valued what I said, which wasn't happening with anyone I knew. And they validated my experience, which I couldn't even understand because I didn't know what I was doing or why. They understood that and validated that for me. They cared about me. That is what got my attention." This was the first time in his life that he had heard men talking about love and spirituality and seen them treating each other with care and kindness. "It was unbelievable. . . . I didn't want to get sober, but I wanted that. Then, I wanted that *and* I wanted to get sober." When the small group of men on his unit stayed up late to talk, it was the first time Marv had ever felt a deep sense of affinity and community. After four weeks, he was now scared to leave. "It was twenty-eight days back then, and that was it. There was no follow up of any kind for a seventeen-year-old in Rochester, Minnesota. They told me to go to AA. This is the only thing, this is it. There wasn't anything else."

Stewartville didn't have an AA group, so Marv just headed back to high school and back into his family, home, and routines. He was told not to hang out with his old friends. He tried. But the people who didn't use drugs didn't want to hang out with him; they had heard the rumors and the gossip about where he had been. Parents did the same, and Marv felt isolated and ostracized. He couldn't last long like this. Within days, he decided it would be fine to go to a concert in the Twin Cities. He got tickets to the Marshall Tucker Band and called his old friend Dave. While Dave was driving, drinking, and smoking pot, Marv sat in the passenger seat explaining his treatment at Hazelden, and how maybe Dave needed help, too. Dave didn't buy it, but he didn't rebuke Marv for whatever he needed to do. At the concert, they met up with some friends. Marv recalled, "There's pot being passed up and down the row and a joint comes by, and I took it and smoked it. I took some, and then more, and then had some beer, and I don't know what else. I was just right back to where I was, just like that. Not any thought about it." He began using heavily after that night and tried again briefly to hide it and to make good grades; he failed at that, too, and didn't graduate from high school. That summer, his dad got him a good job, but he never showed up. His parents kicked him out, disowned him, and said they would not be paying for college. He packed up his Volkswagen and moved to Rochester.

IBM and the Mayo Clinic were the biggest employers in Rochester at the time, and since IBM was out of the question due to his dad, he applied for a janitor position at a lab at Mayo. When he got called for an interview, they told him to go to the cardiovascular research lab. He was interviewed and hired by a world-famous physiologist, David Donald, as a lab technician for his research team. As Marv soon learned, people from all over the world came to work under Dr. Donald and Dr. John Shepherd, the two directors of the lab, who couldn't have been more different from one another. Shepherd was fastidiously clean and always wore a suit. Donald lived out in the woods by himself, never dressed up, and always wore a white lab coat with old shoes he had taped together. At the time, Marv sported long hair, so he wondered if he'd been hired by Donald to give "Shepherd a hard time with this hippie drug-addict kid."[37] His employer did not know about his drug use, but he wondered about his hiring nonetheless. Marv still struggled with substance use and missed a week of work before his three-month probationary period, but he loved this job from the first moment he walked into the lab. He ended up learning a tremendous amount about physiology, assisted in experiments and surgeries, and was soon included in the group discussions of researchers and fellows who gathered weekly for lab meetings. When they noticed his intellectual curiosity, the question of college came up. What did he think about going on to school someday?

Marv and his parents were estranged for about two years, but at one point early on in his time at Mayo, he was having a hard time dealing with cocaine use. He called his dad, who agreed to meet him and talk. It turned out that Marv's father had become involved in a new adolescent drug and alcohol center called Sunrise. He was on the board. He introduced Marv to a counselor who encouraged him to attend meetings at their center in Rochester. Despite his misgivings, he really didn't want to lose his job at Mayo, so he went, but remembered the advice from Hazelden and chose to attend AA instead. Three guys over seventy were at the first meeting he attended. He went only once a week, which Marv assumed was the norm in the 1970s. Since leaving treatment and moving to Rochester, he had never been to an AA meeting. He kept going, and attendance at the meeting grew to include women and men in a variety of professions. "Because I was so young, there was a lot of parenting in addition to everything else that goes on in AA." He had made supportive and sober friends, learned how to fly-fish, and moved in with his high school girlfriend, Linda, his wife to this day. He felt better than he ever had.

One Sunday he didn't go to his usual meeting, and then that Monday he used. Six months sober and he used again—he still doesn't know exactly why. The three original old-timers of the meeting had died within those six months. He missed them. Maybe that was part of it, maybe not. "This is the worst day of my life. Six months and I am no longer sober, and to me, I tried treatment and that didn't work; my own efforts got me two weeks, and AA got me six months. That doesn't work either. And they didn't tell me anything else that I could do. . . . I think that I am hopeless. I did as much cocaine as I possibly could, more than any other day in my life. I didn't even notice it because the pain was so bad of losing that [sobriety], of what I had." He remembered a guy named John at the meeting, someone he admired, a thirty-something father with five years' sobriety. He called him up. They met that afternoon at his son's Pee Wee football practice. Marv told him what he had done, how he had failed. John said, "You know Marv, AA works fine, you just haven't started." And then he said, "You come to the meetings, but you're not working the Steps, you're not reading the books, you're not talking to anybody, you're not sharing yourself with anybody. You need to start doing that. AA works fine. I'm proof." Marv said, okay, and then did exactly what John told him to do.

For the next five years, Marv filled out a worksheet every night to keep track of his assets and liabilities. This process is part of what people in AA and NA refer to as Step Ten work. Step Four is "Made a searching and fearless moral inventory of ourselves," and Step Ten continues that reflective process: "Continued to take personal inventory and when we were wrong promptly admitted it." Marv described what John gave him. "This sheet was a ten-step inventory sheet. So, it had thirty-one days across the top and all of these columns and rows, that had on one side a list of liabilities, and the other side, a list of assets. The liabilities were like laziness, dishonesty . . . they were listed there, like twenty or twenty-five adjectives. And then the assets were their opposites, basically." Because he was so scared that he would relapse, he filled it out every night, changing it up a little when the assets and liabilities became too rote. In the first year, he remembered that he put an X by "dishonesty" every day. This was hard for me to imagine, so I asked, "What were you being dishonest about *every* day?"

> Everything. I just couldn't be honest. I was so dishonest for so long that it was almost a ritual. Most of the time it didn't even make sense to be dishonest anymore, but I did. So, John, he kept

telling me, "You know Marv, this is an honesty program." And that's all he would say. And finally, I realized . . . that I am always dishonest. . . . He was an ideal person for me. He never confronted me. I would tell him something going on in my life, like I'm having trouble with my girlfriend Linda, or whatever. And he would just tell me some story from his life. It would always have some connection to what I was talking about.

Marv appreciated that John was not prescriptive or overly analytical. John had a daughter who was only a couple of years younger than Marv, so he credits John for some exceptional parenting skills as well. He led by example.

One day at the lab, Marv received one of those lined, manila office envelopes, and someone had written on the addressee line, "Dr. Marvin Seppala." He told me he still has it, an old interoffice envelope. I immediately thought of it as being a kind of talisman for the future then but now a memento from the past. Reflecting a bit more deeply on this memory, he said, of that time, "I am being influenced by science in the lab, but also by people and caring. In AA, I am being influenced by the Twelve Steps and love and spirituality. . . . My life grows in all of those spheres."

We laughed when he said he only applied to one undergraduate school—St. Olaf, a small liberal arts college in Northfield, Minnesota, surrounded by corn fields. He sees now how he put his future in the hands of one admissions office. Fortunately, he was accepted. His first day of college was on his one-year sobriety anniversary. He described the partying all around him, but he continued to drive to Rochester for his weekly AA meeting on Sundays. He immediately told his dorm mates about his sobriety and the reason for it; they took it seriously and kept an eye out for him. "They were just really practical. [They would say,] 'That makes sense, Marv, you shouldn't do that.'" He and these friends still get together. They laugh about how St. Olaf advertised that it was a dry campus, as there was alcohol and pot readily available, and how they always had to watch out for Marv's safety.

Marv and Linda married, and they finished their undergraduate degrees at Drake University in Iowa. Marv applied to Mayo—again, one place—for medical school. He was accepted, and by his second year thought he would specialize in cardiac surgery, given his years of work as a lab technician. He was excited about this until the start of clinical rotations, when he realized how many people were in the hospital due to medical issues created by underlying alcohol and drug problems. "We weren't diagnosing it, we weren't writing it down, even. We were not giving referrals; we were not giving consultations. Nothing you would normally do for an illness did we do." After his one-month psychiatry rotation, he found an attraction to the field that he did not expect, "and it was a gateway to work in addiction." It was 1984. He remembered telling a couple of the attending physicians that he planned to go into psychiatry and specialize in addiction. They all said, in one way or another, "You're throwing away a good career in medicine."[38]

As a few other addiction medicine doctors told me during our interviews, this was a common response. Even though he applied to residencies on both coasts, trying to get away from the Midwest, Marv ended up going to the University of Minnesota Hospitals. His disappointment about not being placed in programs on the coasts vanished. He realized that this was where he belonged. They had an addiction medicine fellowship program, and he was able to work alongside Dr. Joe Westermeyer, head of the Veterans Administration hospital and world-renowned for his work with Southeast Asian opium users, refugees, and war-traumatized populations. He also worked with Dr. Mark Willenbring, an alcohol and addiction medicine specialist, and John Brantner, a doctor who studied thanatology (death and suicide) and was part of the group who developed the MMPI, the Minnesota Multiphasic Personality Inventory. From another mentor at the VA, Dick Heilman, he learned that group therapy "was as important as surgery, and you can't interrupt it." Marv trained at a time when psychoanalysis was still a major aspect of psychiatry, but the biologic psychiatrists were rapidly trying to change the field to focus more on medications and neurophysiology than talk therapy, where both were at the university and "warring with each other, basically." New medications for psychiatric illnesses, depression, and anxiety were coming on the market then. Prozac was approved for use while Marv was a resident in the mid-1980s. He felt fortunate that he learned about these new drugs while also being trained in psychoanalysis. After that time, many programs stopped offering that training in favor of biomedicine, leaving talk therapy to the psychologists.[39]

One of Seppala's underlying motivations for becoming a psychiatrist and studying addiction science was that he wanted to go back to work at Hazelden. He felt that his own positive experience with the

Twelve Steps, his grounding in lab science and medicine, and now his psychiatry specialization gave him skills to integrate all three in order to help people suffering from substance use disorders and other mental health crises. He soon learned that Hazelden had no openings and that they, like most treatment centers, did not have a psychiatrist on staff. They contracted with psychiatric consultants on a very limited basis. Hazelden did employ full-time psychologists, though, since it was primarily a psychotherapy-oriented program. For clients on medication, the services of a psychiatrist were needed on a very limited basis for prescription refills and medication adjustments.

Over several years and moves between Washington, Oregon, and Minnesota, Seppala pieced together a work schedule with different organizations and addiction treatment programs, but he always felt called back to Hazelden. After a short stint there in 1995 as the first medical director, when Hazelden had decided they should hire a medical director, he left because he had no guidance or mandate to do anything of any substance. He and his family went back to Oregon for good. In 2001, Hazelden bought an addiction treatment center there, Springbrook, and Marv was hired again to be the medical director in charge of Hazelden's seventeen sites in nine states.

By this time, he wanted to conduct research for evidence-based studies about the Minnesota Model, also known as TSF, Twelve Step Facilitation, but he was up against entrenched forces that limited changes to the clinical program. He "held on" from 2001 until 2007. The counselor training program was old and established, but "without the academics, there was not a learning culture at Hazelden." Having come from Mayo and the University of Minnesota, he knew that so much exciting research and innovation was in the works for addiction treatment. Things were changing rapidly. Suboxone was approved in 2007. Pain pill and heroin use was on a precipitous rise. Marv was incredibly frustrated and said so in his resignation letter. Before he left Hazelden, now for the third time, he recalled, "I thought to myself, we really ought to consider this medicine—the only one for opioid use disorder."[40]

He returned to Portland and began working on how to integrate Suboxone and naltrexone (at that time used for alcohol use disorder, not yet for opioid) into an outpatient, home-based, detox treatment model. He lectured about the opioid crisis and the new medicines available. He said that it felt as if no one was listening. He worked with this new program and others for the next two years. Then he told me that a colleague of his now jokes that Hazelden has been his "Hotel California." What a great analogy, on so many levels. We laughed. And then, while I was still giggling, he told me he returned to Hazelden again in 2009 as their chief medical officer. He has been there ever since, commuting to Center City as needed, but working from the Springbrook location in Oregon. Now he was especially anxious to get started with his idea for implementing a medication-based, Twelve Step–guided program for clients with opioid use disorder similar to the one he began testing in Portland. He had to convince the board members of its promise. He gathered supporters—the CEO, Mark Mishek, and a beloved priest, Father Michael Connell, as well as other board members—and in 2011, the board approved the new program for use at Hazelden.

They named it COR-12. COR stands for Comprehensive Opioid Response, and the number twelve signifies the Twelve Step–focused programming.[41] By January 2012, he was gathering a clinical team from all of Hazelden's sites to get the plan implemented. One interested counselor nervously asked him if it was a good career move, since associating with medications could be dicey if the program didn't work. Marv explained, "I had to convince people of its worth, so I thought I would just use the literature" and the overdose death data. By that, he meant the studies on medications for opioid use disorders. After that, most of his colleagues admitted it was hard to refute the evidence of the drugs' efficacy. To establish support from the old-guard AA staff, he enlisted Fred Ulmquist, a respected, nationally known speaker for Hazelden. Fred teaches like a professor, according to Marv, and he used *The Big Book* and the Twelve Traditions of AA to argue that AA literature actually says that medical care and medications are private and between an individual and their doctor.

To get everyone at Hazelden on board, and in the spirit of full disclosure, Marv, Fred, and Scott, the counselor who had previously worried about it being a good career move, developed a community forum where they each presented aspects of the new program and took ample time for questions and concerns. More than one hundred staff attended the first of these sessions. Marv spoke first and described how the medications worked. Scott's presentation followed Marv's. He asked the audience, "How many people here have had a client die of an overdose after leaving treatment?" Marv said at least 75 percent of the hands went up. Of course, there were overlaps among these, but each staff member whose hand was raised had known and interacted with that client. He recalled of that moment, "You could hear a pin drop." They still expected hard questions but "got softball question after softball question." Then one of their most conservative, AA-focused counselors stood up. Marv girded himself. She said:

> My daughter went to residential treatment three times for heroin, relapsed after each treatment right away, could not get sober until she started taking Suboxone. And now she has been sober three years, she's part of my family again; she now takes care of her children and I don't have to anymore; she has a job, and she is doing wonderfully.

As he spoke to me, Marv looked as astonished as he must have that day. He was elated. He explained more.

> And no one knew. She hadn't told anyone. . . . We couldn't have asked for anything better to say, and it was just from the most unlikely person in the room, just this *Big Book*–thumping woman who no one ever thought would ever support this. And it was the most incredible description of the utility of this medication that you could ever hear. And her daughter went to AA, right? And took the medicine!

His new program was not out of hot water just yet, though. They were "lambasted by other treatment programs," and a prominent AA person in the Twin Cities criticized both him and the organization for "turning our back on our entire heritage, ruining the treatment field, and ruining Hazelden." Within the same month, he was also told by a St. Paul doctor that they weren't giving clients *enough* medication. The criticisms from both sides went on for a while, but he persisted in his belief that COR-12 would help many more people recover for the long-term. "We saw the utility of a residential stay for stabilization, followed by long-term outpatient, during which people could transition from professional care to self-care over months and years, if it was necessary. And it gave us the opportunity to maintain involvement and support ongoing use of medications, and ultimately, if they wanted to get off, we could be there to help them with that and insure continued support."

The first group of COR-12 clients continued to meet with each other for two years, with all of the same people alive and present. They were on medication and attending Twelve Step meetings. Hazelden conducted another study from 2013 to 2017 with 259 participants of COR-12 to assess the program's effectiveness.[42] The clients had been given a choice of medications—Vivitrol, Suboxone, or none—and their choices broke down into about equal thirds. There were three deaths among that group. One had used Suboxone and two Vivitrol. None of the "no meds" clients had passed away. Even Marv was surprised by these low numbers.

It was unlike me and even antithetical to my style as an oral historian, but I pressed Dr. Seppala quite a bit in our second interview, particularly regarding the effectiveness of COR-12. I thought about all the families I knew who had lost loved ones, and I mentioned Ryan Lewis, who died of an overdose in 2014 at a Hazelden-run sober house. Marv could see where I was headed, and I didn't even have to ask before he acknowledged that they still don't have adequate knowledge of these deaths. "I want to study a thousand of our patients with opioid use disorder and look at all of their deaths through the Social Security Death Index, because [it] has gotten really much better at defining death by overdose." Studying when people died by overdose post-treatment and what medications they were on, though difficult, is imperative.

To his credit, he wasn't going to take all the blame and gently reminded me that "every single treatment program in the country is dealing with this." Yes, true. I knew that, I just hoped for more accountability from the industry as a whole on this issue. Most treatment programs don't conduct outcome studies, and they don't do follow-up studies with their clients. They are not required to. They track the numbers of people who come in for treatment, what their main drug is, and how long they stay. Marv recalled his frustration in the years before COR-12 when he was speaking at professional conferences. "I was talking about death and overdose at every single discussion that I had about it, because it is so necessary to the discussion. If you are going to change your whole model, you have to have a good reason. There is no better reason. And nobody would engage in a conversation about that." I asked if these were just Twelve Step programs he was referring to, and he said he was talking about everyone, addiction medicine doctors included. He admitted that at recent American Society of Addiction Medicine conferences, people had begun to talk about death rates, but he suspects that the lag was because drug treatment staff had so rarely experienced the deaths of clients that they just didn't know what to do when the opioid epidemic began its rampage. And still, there is no governing body that tracks and follows post-treatment outcomes. "It's ridiculous. And so, if you assume that everyone is doing great and put on your website that 90 percent are abstinent at one year, you can't look and see who died." He wants more studies, more research, more accountability.

I always closed interviews with physicians by asking what they felt most gratified about in their work, and if they could change anything about addiction treatment, what would that be? Marv, like all the others, wanted addiction treatment available to everyone for as long as they needed it, and it needed to be affordable and easily accessible. The second time we spoke, having clocked five hours over two interviews, he closed by recalling how little professional or peer support he had when he left treatment at age seventeen. He wants addiction treatment to be long-term and multifaceted, with many kinds of support mechanisms available for as long as needed. And he wants it to be evidence-based, research-oriented, and full of loving-kindness. The last word there is mine, because after I turned off the recording device, Marv told me he was working on writing a book about love. Of course he was.

CHAPTER 4

Women of Substance

Harm Reduction in Minnesota

For most of my life, I thought that the term "overdose" implied certain death. I remember hearing about celebrity overdoses in my childhood and teenage years—Marilyn Monroe, Jim Morrison, Elvis Presley, John Belushi, among others—so in my limited knowledge, overdose meant the person had died. I did not know someone could survive an overdose. After my daughter's nonfatal overdose, I discovered that I was not alone in my misunderstanding of the term. Now I know that many people survive opioid overdoses, but when I first used the word, almost everyone had a hesitant look followed by an awkward follow-up question: *Did she survive?* Maybe there is something inherently ambiguous about the word "overdose," situated as it is on that fine line between life and death, between surviving or not surviving. And that sticky stigma always seemed to attach itself to these conversations; whether visible or more elusive, it was always there.

This early memory of the fatal shame of "overdose" would now confirm the fine line I frequently traversed in all kinds of experiences. While we were huddled in the medical intensive care unit for eleven days wondering if Madeleine would regain the ability to breathe on her own, I overheard teaching doctors and residents refer to her as "an OD." Although I later learned it is common for medical staff to use such shorthand, the callousness of the term made me cringe. Did they name other patients "a car accident" or "a stroke," as they passed their rooms? The sting of that moment was softened only because my sister, herself a physician, stopped the group of residents in the hall and asked them to please consider using a patient's name when family are present on their rounds. This was just the first glimmer of my understanding of how deeply entrenched stigma is in all aspects of

our society. Its pervasiveness had remained elusive to me until suddenly I noticed it everywhere.

Once I could no longer unsee stigma, I began to recognize how I
had been stigmatizing drug users through fear born of ignorance that
then led to moral and ethical judgments. Fearing and then judging
something we don't understand is an easy out that makes ignorance
about that thing easier to maintain. Hard drug use truly scared me,
and so it seemed obvious that I should also fear people who used those
drugs. Aside from the "logic" born of ingrained stereotypes, the biggest challenge was understanding why someone would use hard drugs
in the first place, and then why they couldn't "just stop." I had no personal experience with drug use. None. And I was definitely one of the
few kids in the entire country during the early 1980s for whom Nancy
Reagan's "Just Say No" campaign actually worked. Reflecting on the
failure of that particular policy approach, my inborn nature was most
likely the reason—I have always been risk averse.[1]

Since parenting tests nearly every aspect of one's being, understanding drug use and its varied degrees of risk became one of my
biggest challenges—I rose to it, but not without a struggle. In the circles of parents and professionals I knew, quitting all drug and alcohol use definitively was the only answer; the Minnesota Model of drug
treatment predominated, and so I assumed that must be what worked;
using illegal drugs meant there would likely be criminal charges and
perhaps incarceration. Most, if not all, family support groups based on
the Twelve Steps of AA supported the Minnesota treatment model. I
would eventually learn about methadone clinics, but only one or two
people I knew of had successful recoveries on methadone, so it seemed
like a long shot. Once while visiting a suburban methadone clinic, I was
shocked and confused when I saw a staff person hand a brown paper
bag of clean syringes to a potential client. How was that helping them
stop using? When drug use is believed to be the reason people get into
trouble with addiction and the law, why on earth would anyone justify
spending time and resources helping people continue to use drugs? I
was completely uninformed.

I knew about Narcan (naloxone), the opioid antidote, from my
earlier experience with a group of mothers affiliated with the Steve
Rummler Hope Network, but I didn't understand how it was connected to syringe exchanges, clean needles, and the grassroots phi-

losophy of harm reduction until a few years later.[2] Although legal efforts to increase access to naloxone were on the rise, the phrase "harm reduction" was not included because it had a negative connection to something edgier and perhaps scarier: needle exchanges for injection drug users.[3] Given the stigma associated with drug users, it was a smart rhetorical strategy to not use that term and simply refer to naloxone as "a life-saving tool" that allowed someone overdosing the chance to live and then, hopefully, get into a treatment program. The diligent work of the Steve Rummler Hope Network in Minnesota, following a growing national model, must be credited with helping to change state laws that kept Narcan away from people who needed it the most: the general public, injection drug users, and police officers; but it was not publicized as being part of a harm reduction philosophy. Even using the term "harm reduction" was taboo in the mid-2010s because of long-standing stigma about drug users and harm reduction's connection to the most marginalized of them: the poor, people of color, and the unhoused.[4]

People who inject drugs (and those who work to keep them safe) have been taking care of each other with needle exchanges since the late 1980s. They sourced underground naloxone. They coined the term "harm reduction" and expanded on its use, applications, and potential.[5] They practiced a philosophy of respect, safety, and care while the War on Drugs incarcerated and devastated entire communities. Their approach is best explained by a handout made by Edith Springer, one of the founders of harm-reduction practices: "Show client unconditional regard and caring. Acknowledge her or his intrinsic worth and dignity. . . . Be mindful of the stages of change. . . . Any reduction in harm is a step in the right direction."[6] Harm reduction is about building relationships and offering support in a nonjudgmental way. One Minneapolis harm reduction activist, Lee Hertel, described it eloquently.

> It's everything intangible. It's everything that makes people walk taller and straighter and maybe just a little bit cockier. That would be the respect that I afford everybody, the dignity, the trust, the love, the belief, and a total non-judgmental attitude. That, I think, is equally as important as the actual physical prevention of the transmission of disease, HIV, hepatitis C,

hepatitis B, any other type of blood-borne virus, hep A, hep D. . . . When you feel like you have someone who loves you, who cares about you, you're going to treat yourself better.[7]

An earlier group of trailblazing women in Minnesota provided Narcan via a doctor's prescription to drug users at a needle exchange in Minneapolis twenty years before the Steve Rummler Hope Foundation began its well-publicized efforts. Through a surprising coincidence, I found Rae Eden Frank on an online Narcotics Anonymous "Speakers List" and set up an interview with her, not having any idea she was the daughter of Kathie Simon Frank, the St. Paul Nar-Anon group founder. Rae became a harm-reduction advocate in Minneapolis in the late 1990s when she moved with her young daughter back to Minnesota from an increasingly precarious, isolated life on the West Coast where she struggled with injection drugs, despite some time in residential treatment.[8] Once back home, she stopped using drugs, reenrolled in college, and got her life back on track. Although she had personal success with a Twelve Step program, her career interest upon her return home was to work in harm-reduction services. "When I came back to Minnesota and I started connecting with some of my old friends, many of them were dead through either overdose or suicide. One hundred percent of [the surviving friends] had hepatitis C. . . . I found out about a needle exchange that was hiring. It was called Women with a Point." She connected me with Sue Purchase, cofounder of the organization. "Sue would probably love to talk to you. She is delightful. . . . She's got a ton of historical stuff with heroin use in the Twin Cities and establishing a needle exchange."

A few months later, I sat in my living room listening, riveted, to Sue Purchase, a former injection drug user who had been taking care of other drug users, particularly women, long before pain pills and heroin-laced fentanyl became a public health crisis. Her life story and the act of sharing it was moving, provocative, and transformative for both of us. In my search for new ways to understand and analyze how our country treats people with a substance use disorder, she confirmed my growing ambivalence about a person needing to hit "rock bottom" and then adhere to "abstinence-only" treatment methods. Before we met each other that year, I knew of no other preventative model. In a country dominated by the abstinence philosophy of AA, it's little wonder that I had not the slightest understanding of what needle exchanges were, much less what they accomplished in humanitarian and public health circles.

Sue Purchase introduced me to the origin story of harm reduction—a once derided but now back-in-favor pragmatic social movement that has usually been in the shadows of conversations about drug use, despite its positive, preventative health impacts.[9] She generously welcomed me into the local, national, and global harm-reduction community and connected me with people who care for and work on behalf of folks who are among the most shunned, mistreated, and cast aside in our society. Purchase is little in stature, but she is a mighty force of tenacity, courage, and conviction. She crossed her legs and sank back into my couch with a familiarity I recognized and appreciated. I wondered if we might become friends.

After our interview, Sue introduced me to one of her closest childhood friends, Deb Holman, a street outreach worker who assists people who lack housing, whether they are living on the streets or camping in the woods surrounding Duluth, Minnesota. Sue and Deb's lifelong friendship and intertwined life stories came to embody both the history and humanity of harm reduction for me. To listen to the stories of Sue Purchase and Deb Holman is to discover how two exceptionally resilient, caretaking, and community-oriented women thrived in spite of the chaos and traumas they lived through. Their lives took different paths, but their commitment to helping others using a harm-reduction philosophy remained in tandem. Both have experience with chaotic and managed substance use, to differing degrees. Deb went to inpatient drug treatment many times in different places around the state, and Sue has never been once. "I could go to school and do other things and just work my way through it. Treatment wasn't a necessity for me."[10] The arc of their lifelong friendship is a microhistory of drug-treatment protocol and harm-reduction practices from the 1970s to the present. Their early life histories and experiences in young adulthood paved the way for the work to which they later committed themselves.

Sue Jurvelin was born in 1959 and grew up in northern Minnesota, primarily in and around the town of Cloquet. One of six children, she described her family's economic status as "working poor," though she acknowledged that her father's job as a manager at the Cloquet Co-Op Store and later at Potlatch paper mill had provided enough income for her mother to stay at home, though not comfortably. She vividly remembered her mother, Dorothy, "scrabbling for money, always worried about money." Sue's father, Charlie, often drank heavily after work, so when he came home and passed out, she watched her mother go through his wallet to see what was left. Sue's family qualified for school lunches under Lyndon B. Johnson's War on Poverty program, and she remembered the lunch program's special blue and yellow tickets.[11] "There was some sort of order to the tickets, but I remember the shame. I hated it. I hated using them." This small memory with a big emotion led her directly to a much harder one.

> Growing up I always felt like everybody in town knew about my
> house, which was fairly true. [My father] was a drinker and he
> was violent. I grew up [on] Carleton Avenue . . . one of the main
> streets in Cloquet. I always felt like we were on display for all of
> the dysfunction and violence and drinking that happened there.
> Always a lot of shame related to it.

Sue's father was physically abusive with her mother and every child in the family, but she remembered him as being less violent with her. Her mother did not drink at all but may have had mental health issues; Sue remembered her as not being supportive, often pitting her children against each other. "She knew divide and conquer really well."

Sue learned early on that she could take refuge at her grandmother's house in the nearby town of Floodwood, Minnesota. "From the time I was really little I'd write to my grandma. . . . I would ask her if I could come stay with her. It would just be arranged. I don't remember exactly how I got a stamp or if I figured out you didn't need to necessarily have a stamp on the envelope. I knew where the mailbox was on the corner." Her uncle would come to Cloquet and pick her up, and she would stay with her grandmother for however many days they had arranged. When she got older, she would hop on the Greyhound bus. "I started out really young just taking care of business. I've always known that I could only depend on myself.

Dorothy divorced Charlie when Sue was in third grade, and then a couple of years later she moved to Oregon with her three youngest children, Sue among them. The relocation did not work out, and they moved back into the same house in Cloquet six months later. Her now estranged father was supposed to move out of the house upon their return but lingered, and two weeks later, he died of a stroke in the living room. The ground was too cold to bury her dad when he died, so "they kept him somewhere until the ground thawed in the spring." Sue doesn't recall much of that winter, except for the relief of having him gone. "I didn't have to worry about his violence any longer." The year was a formative one in terms of her own consciousness. "When I think about myself, it was Susie who moved to Oregon. I was always known as Susie, as a little girl. My mother would always talk about how Susie was so docile and so calm." She laughed out loud describing when they returned to Minnesota: "That's when 'A Boy Named Sue' showed up! My alter ego. I love Johnny Cash." Her brothers played his music and so she knew the song well. "I had to be a badass to survive. If I was going to be sweet and docile, I wasn't going to make it."

Even being tougher than most, sixth grade was still hard—the move, a new school, coming back, and then her father's death. One good thing about that school year was that she met Connie. "She had older siblings and a fucked-up family life, too. . . . There were some older girls in the neighborhood, and we started smoking cigarettes and drinking. My older brother was married and had a little girl and I used to babysit. I used to steal their cigarettes. . . . I would [bring] booze to school in a baby food jar." The summer between sixth and seventh grade, the two friends got into a little more serious trouble: they were caught shoplifting in Duluth. The police were involved, and then somehow the school was involved, too, because later that fall she had to visit with a guidance counselor. She liked him but felt confused by some of the things he said, like when he referred to her as being a survivor. "I remember sitting there thinking, 'What the fuck does that mean? How do you know that about me? What's going on? What do you know that I don't know? What does that mean? What am I surviving?'" Despite his good intentions to connect with her somehow, she withdrew. "This is my life. I am twelve. I don't have insights. It made me so uncomfortable."

Cloquet elementary schools fed into one junior high school, and there Sue met several more girls who also became lifelong friends. Debbie Holman and her close friend Mary came from Sacred Heart Catholic School; friends Lisa, Robin, Connie, and a few others made the core group about ten. The school system had implemented something called modular scheduling, a short-lived, 1960s educational experiment where many twenty-minute "mods" made up a student's day, and they moved from class to class frequently. Sue remembered the feeling of autonomy and independence that came with it, as well as the freedom to get into trouble. They began cajoling marijuana from an older brother of one of the girls, and so he nicknamed them the "Weedweevils." The girls then gave each other nicknames to go along with their new club: Mad Dog, Crazy Fry Brain, Weehelvie, and Susie Monster. Before school, this group of girls would gather at Mary's home—her mother left early for work—and they would smoke pot. "We'd get really high. Then we'd go to school. We had a presence. We were rascals and fun and outrageous and didn't give a shit. We weren't shy. . . . We had no fear."

The pot smoking during school days led to dropping acid at school parties. Getting drugs from older kids was simple, and the girls were "resourceful," as Sue put it. They could easily leave school. One day they left to smoke pot on the grounds of a nearby church. "We're back there getting high. Somebody reported us so the principal comes from one way, the assistant principal from the other way. We're caught and suspended from school. My mother was pissed." The three-day suspension was an in-school punishment. Their drug use continued to escalate.

In ninth grade, Sue left home to live with her brother, his wife, and small child because the situation with her mother was getting hard and not just because of Sue's "wild" behavior. Besides being an avid letter writer, she had kept a diary for years. Her mother found it, read it, and then started to use the information against her. Recalling this, Sue exhaled, "I didn't write after that." Although her brother's house provided more structure in terms of family life, responsibilities, and respect, she also had more freedom to do what she wanted, including smoking and drinking with them. The Weedweevils became even more emboldened around this time, bucking a town and a culture that to them was behind the times. "You don't talk about stuff—it's northern Minnesota. It's the sixties, the early seventies. Things might be changing, things might be becoming more liberal but not in northern Minnesota. There's tradition." From her perspective as a fifty-something woman looking back on her fifteen-year-old self, much of their behavior was about having fun and being empowered, about taking up space in the world and claiming their own experiences as young women who had the right to the same things young men did, and that included using drugs. "Girls were not supposed to be wild and out of hand and rebellious and have a club that is all about getting high and getting over. We did. It was like, 'Fuck you. You think we shouldn't do this? Well, we're going to show you what we can do.' We didn't care. We had fun."

And then one of them got sent away. Sue recalled this moment with both tears, anger, and frustration over the powerlessness and defiance she felt as a teenage girl in a messed-up world. "We wanted to be badasses, 'hoods' they'd call us. Debbie gets sent away. I remember there was conversation around that. I don't know how we knew what we knew. . . . She's gone for a long time. It is a therapeutic community. We were fourteen. Oh my God. It's Debbie's story to tell. . . . It was intense."

Deb Holman was fourteen the first time she was admitted to a Duluth inpatient drug-treatment program. Two days later, she and another teen girl ran away from the facility, but ended up back in a detox, where they again ran away, in their pajamas, in the dark of the night. She doesn't remember if she was officially "committed" by child protective services but does remember being assigned a social worker and sent to a group home for "wayward ladies" as she called it, the Booth Brown House in St. Paul, where she spent about six months.[12] She eventually got into trouble there for using drugs and drinking. After that incident, she ended up at St. Mary's Hospital in a drug-treatment program. She couldn't recall the name of the particular kind of treatment model used but described it vividly.

> It was very confrontational. . . . You had to sign a contract. If you left the program and wanted to come back, you had to be willing to sacrifice something. Some people cut their hair or shaved their head. Then at that point they made people wear signs and stuff, too. I was fourteen or fifteen I think, fourteen probably, and I wore this sign that said, "I'm a lying, cheating, slippery, slick junkie." I wish I had a picture of it. Part of my thought is that, "Well, you made me one." . . . You made me wear this sign, so I became a self-fulfilling prophecy. Then the other part of me knows there's addiction in my family.[13]

What Deb experienced was a program based on the therapeutic community (TC) model, the second generation of treatment practices that originated with Synanon in the 1960s, a form of treatment based on the idea that it was possible to change the negative and childish behavior of "hardcore" drug users permanently and authentically, through confrontation and ridicule in an intense, "familial" residential therapy environment.[14] One of the main tools was shame, which was deployed in a variety of ways to break a person down in order to build them back up. From the 1970s to the mid-1980s, TC programming became well established in jails, youth detention centers, prisons, hospital programs, and private treatment centers.

When she graduated from high school in 1978, Deb had been to treatment three times in three different places around the state: a Duluth treatment center she couldn't recall the name of, St. Mary's Riverside Hospital in Minneapolis, and Willmar State Hospital, in Willmar, Minnesota. The third hospital, as earlier chapters noted, was one of the founding institutions for the Minnesota Model of drug treatment and was on the forefront of what it became those decades and following.

One of the first things Deb told me when we met at a coffee shop in Duluth was that her family has a history of alcoholism and addiction issues. She referred to her grandpa as a "mean drunk" who committed suicide when she was in second grade; her dad was a "weekend drunk," and her mom was "super stable, obviously probably codependent, just one of those people that everyone loved, just because that's just the way she was." When she started "acting out" in junior high—getting in trouble for drinking, skipping school, fights at home—she would blame it on her dad, and yet, looking back on it, she was confident that she did not really have what she called a "bad" home life. Her mom was emotionally stable, and her dad worked, though he did get drunk on the weekends and was known to throw things. They divorced when she was eighteen, and Deb, as the oldest of four siblings, has sometimes blamed herself. "I always felt like I kind of pushed that. I kind of felt bad. As I look back on it now, I was a little brat to my parents. . . . Why was I like that?" Over the years, she has also searched her memory for something, for some clue, to explain her struggle with substance use, but nothing traumatic has ever surfaced. She attributes it now to genetics and family history. "I was one of those [people] that would use whatever. . . . I know I have the addictive personality."[15]

The summer after high school graduation, Deb moved to the Twin Cities, rented a small apartment, and got a job at a photo store. She hung out with Cloquet friends and continued to drink and use drugs, and vividly recalled the sudden popularity of cocaine in the early 1980s. Due to her early experiences with drug treatment, Deb knew how to use employee assistance programs, health insurance, and the treatment system whenever she became aware of how her responsibilities to her job were starting to suffer because of her drug use. Keeping a job was always a priority for her. "Every time that I started to get to the point where maybe things were getting out of control or 'I'm like missing work now,' the answer I would always think would be, 'Go to treatment.' Now looking back, I don't think that was the answer. I think that was ingrained in me because of my experience." Even so, Deb always made great connections in treatment and fondly remembered some of those people and places as we talked. Although she never stayed completely abstinent from substance use, she thrived socially while living in treatment and sober housing. Eventually, she knew that she'd probably never give up smoking pot, and that alcohol was actually the most dangerous substance for her. Drinking quickly led to heavier, more dangerous drug use, so she avoided getting drunk. She did not learn this in treatment but in life—the way the majority of people learn to temper and even stop dangerous or chaotic substance use. This kind of self-knowledge and self-regulation is integral to the goals of harm reduction, but she didn't know that yet.

For a time after high school graduation, Deb and Sue both lived in Minneapolis. In fact, six of the original Weedweevils moved to Minneapolis, either temporarily, like Sue, or more long term, like Deb. They spent many nights at Moby's, an infamous bar on Hennepin Avenue in downtown Minneapolis. The bar and the night life on Hennepin, nicknamed "the Midwest Times Square," were featured in a multistory report by well-known Twin Cities local news anchor Dave Moore in 1978. As Moore drives and narrates, the Tom Waits song "The Heart of Saturday Night" opens and closes each segment. Sue's description of downtown at that time mirrors the details of the news segment. The two bars featured, Moby Dick's and the Gay 90's, had a long, lively, sordid history and anchored the series' reporting.[16] Sue became happy and animated when she remembered:

> We would drink in Moby Dick's. . . . It used to be downtown on Hennepin Avenue, down by the Gay 90's and Augie's. . . . [My]

friend Brenda, her older brother Bobby was a gay man. He hung out at the Gay 90's all the time. We had an in with older people continually. At Moby's—that place had a reputation! Downtown Minneapolis in the seventies with pimps and sex workers with big hats with feathers. We were in hog heaven. It was fun. It was entertaining. It was a challenge. It wasn't boring. We never liked to be boring.

When I asked if she ever felt scared or in danger, Sue responded that they "should have been scared." She recounted several stories with her friends when they had been in dangerous and compromising situations that caused trauma of some degree or another: multiple car accidents, older men, sexual assaults. "There were a lot of things that got talked about *after* the fact. Apparently one friend was raped during [a] party. I don't know how the circumstances were talked about. . . . Things weren't really acknowledged. They just went on. We went on . . . the Weedweevils slowly dispersed."

Within a year, Sue and Lisa decided to go on a road trip "out West." As she described it, images of Jack Kerouac's *On the Road* came to mind. They planned to go to Mexico but ran out of money in Arizona after traveling all over the West and Southwest for six weeks. Sue's brother wired them enough money to make their way to Denver, where they could stay with a childhood friend of hers. After a short time, she and Lisa "end up going up the mountain to Summit County" after seeing an ad for employment at Keystone Resort. The area was booming due to new ski resorts and other developments. They initially found office jobs but soon worked as construction laborers helping a foreman move equipment from one unit to another. He allowed them to sleep in the finished units until they had enough money to rent a place. The first place was a rented room on Silver Lane in Silverthorne, Colorado, across from the Mint Saloon, one of Willie Nelson's old haunts. At this memory, Sue smiled broadly and said, "We think we have died and gone to heaven."

Sue met her first husband, Ron, at a party in the Silverthorne area. She was immediately drawn to him. "He's got long hair. I immediately think he is something. He's vegetarian, lives in some old trailer. The mountains are not developed. A lot of people lived with wood stoves for heat, kerosene lamps, vegetarians. Kind of that sort of mountain hippie lifestyle, the Grateful Dead. . . . I just think, 'Oh my God, he's cooler than shit.' I picked up with him." Before long, Sue moved into Ron's trailer. He liked to drink heavily, and he was also an intravenous cocaine user.

While I was listening, I noticed that as she spoke Sue seemed to be remembering the beginning and the end of this relationship all at once. Her demeanor changed quickly but subtly. I anticipated that some kind of trauma would soon be shared, and then sure enough, she said, "It was a violent relationship from the very start." Sue first injected drugs with Ron, part in fascination and part as a way to connect with him emotionally. She learned quickly that using with him made their relationship work more smoothly. When she became pregnant, however, she stopped drinking, using drugs, and smoking. She took mothering seriously.

Not much changed with Ron, though, and his violence escalated, despite her pregnancy. Her trauma is evident in her narrative of one frightening moment:

> There was one time he's got me, I'm on the couch, I'm nine months pregnant. I've got my knees pulled to my chest to the degree that you can in that situation. There's a coffee table that was homemade out of two by fours. Those thick pieces of wood, it's L-shaped. He breaks that table. What I remember is him holding a piece of it over my head. It doesn't connect with me. It's really threatening. I don't really remember then what happened there. I know that I run out of the house and that I'm hiding across the road in the ditch. I don't know what happens after that. I end up leaving Ron. Maybe that incident. Maybe it was the night before my baby shower there was something. I don't really know where I went.

She did go back to Ron and soon gave birth to her first child, Krista, before she turned twenty-one. On her birthday that year, some friends came to their house for a little party. "I remember thinking that for many people that turn twenty-one, they want to go to the bar, because that's the legal drinking age. It wasn't a big deal for me at that point. I'd been in the bar for years. I didn't see the excitement of it." She wasn't drinking or using drugs at all. "I took it seriously. Krista was a tiny baby. I've always loved babies." At some point, she went to the bedroom to breastfeed Krista in her rocking chair. "Ron came in, and he punched me in the face. Punched me in the mouth. I'm not sure why, what my offense was, at that point. It seemed out of the blue. He was remorseful the next day and all of that happy shit that goes along with that. That would just continue."

Sue stayed with Ron for five or six more years, moving to different parts of the newly developing ski resort industry as jobs took them places for his work and his drug-using habits. Ron's drug use eventually manifested into intense paranoia, violence, and mental instability. He carried more than one gun with him at all times. Leaving an abuser is the most dangerous moment for survivors, and though she had contemplated and tried to leave many times, she finally and successfully left Ron when Krista was six and their son Blake was three. The three of them fled for their lives in a quick but long-calculated escape and with the help of friends and family. When Ron discovered she was gone, he followed them by car to Oregon but never caught up with them. Sue's sister flew out to help them drive back to Minneapolis. She stayed with family briefly until she was able to secure Section Eight housing and welfare benefits. Sue and her two children lived on $528.00 a month in the Elliot Park neighborhood of Minneapolis. She connected with social service organizations that helped with single parenting, domestic violence, and childcare.

Ron visited Minneapolis in search of Sue at least once but did not find her. He also never got her new phone number. He would occasionally call Sue's sister and arrange a time to speak with Krista and Blake at Sue's sister's home. On one of those occasions, Sue spoke briefly to Ron and remembered his "crazy talking." A week later, after a sunny day with her children at Lake Nokomis in Minneapolis, her brother called to tell her that Ron had died in a car accident. The story Sue later heard from the driver of the car was that they were on a dark country road, and at one point while she was driving, Ron looked at her, said goodbye, opened the door, and jumped out into the dark.

After his funeral, she remembered feeling numb and still in shock; his death was both a relief and a burden. She now had to begin the process of healing from the impact his violence and addictions had had on her and their children. "It was so life changing. It was a huge relief on so many levels. I remember thinking first and foremost that for sure I was a single parent. . . . Very cut and dried. I didn't have to be afraid. I could come and go. To the degree that would be physically possible, the rest was something else." The rest she referred to had to do with how to process his death, the relationship, and the entire family's trauma. He became a kind of ghost in her life, and although it was a relief to no longer be tied to Ron, she nevertheless felt haunted by him. "I just remember thinking, 'Now the bastard's everywhere.' In some ways there was no containing him. Not being able to sleep and always looking over my shoulder, making sure that he was dead." She knew she needed to understand and commit to breaking the cycle of substance use and mental health issues. She didn't know how exactly to break it, or change it, but she knew it had to happen somehow. "It was just so important to figure out the key. But it's not a nice and neat little tidy package. It doesn't happen like that. I think that I thought if I went to therapy, if I went to school, if I did this, if I did that, I would guard against it. If my kids had a college education, if I had a college education. If I made more money, if I did this, if I did that."

After sharing the entire story of her marriage to Ron and his death, Sue was on the edge of the couch, in what seemed to be a heightened state of alert. Looking at me, she could see that I shared her feelings about it. "It is a scary story, isn't it?"

"So scary," I said.

"I am never real sure if I should be scared or what I should do with it. A pause would be good."

I stopped the recorder. We both took a deep breath. I knew that we had to let the trauma of that hard story fade a bit, to let her decide if she even wanted to continue.

Until the day we met, all that I knew of Sue Purchase's life centered on her work with women, harm reduction, and activism. I could see now that the fire in her to do the work she did came from this place, this desire to help other women who faced challenges like her own. Rather than move away from the danger, she stayed near it and tried to help others. She spoke in the simple present tense when talking about these scary, tragic situations. I understood completely. Recalling traumatic memories can change language, diction, and frame of reference. Experiencing trauma can also guide a person to help others heal, to help others stay safe. This was now her calling.

Over the course of the next several years, Sue went back and forth between Minneapolis and Colorado, working full time, going to school full time, and remarrying. She had a third child, Kelly, with her second husband, but their marriage ended after a couple of years. She finally landed back in Minneapolis where she discovered again that she excelled in college. "Education meant so much for me. It opened up a world that I could never have imagined. It signaled the way out. I did really well. I had a 3.8 the whole way through." She was drawn to classes and research projects that focused on helping women. After Ron died, she volunteered in domestic violence organizations in Minneapolis. "This is where I keep getting hung up. . . . Right in there. That's where I wanted to go."

By "right in there," and "this is where I keep getting hung up," Sue meant the passion in her own personal mission where advocacy around harm reduction, drug use, and women's issues intersected. She volunteered at the Domestic Abuse Program after having received services there when she was trying to untangle her life from Ron's. After he passed away, she stayed connected with DAP as a volunteer. "I used to carry a pager. I'd do on-site visits with women. When there was a domestic and an automatic arrest, then we made contact with the women. That was really, really a powerful experience. It moved me in a different direction. . . . It was harm reduction before I ever even had heard the term."

When she said it that way, I began to realize that harm reduction meant many different things, that it was something that could be applied to a lot of different situations. Thinking about the history of women organizing to end domestic violence as a form of harm reduction opened up a whole new set of possibilities to me. Despite the ongoing and historic efforts to end relationship violence, it doesn't appear to be abating in our culture. Many people still cannot understand how or why women return to dangerous relationships. But an array of services and shelters, education and protective laws have definitely reduced the harm that families in violent crises experience. Helping reform the abusers was part of this history, too, so could stigma against them be reduced through a harm-reduction approach? Did domestic violence perpetrators deserve to be understood and destigmatized? Is the recently named concept of toxic masculinity one way to reframe violence and mitigate harm against victims? The scope of harm reduction widened for me in this moment; I could also see that Sue was someone who lived the tenets of the philosophy deeply, long before even she knew that she was.

Sue first heard of the concept of harm reduction as it related to drug use in an academic setting, ironically, while taking a course at

Minneapolis Community and Technical College. The class read from a textbook series called *Opposing Viewpoints*. This particular book focused on the AIDS crisis, and included a section debating the pros and cons of needle exchanges as a way to mitigate the spread of HIV among intravenous drug users.[17] Sue remembered the "con" article as making her angry at the writer—surely even drug users deserve to be safe from HIV/AIDS, don't they? Some lines of the con essay stand out for their sheer cruelty: "They are society's throwaway people, and they know it . . . junkies are an unattractive, unstable lot. The likelihood that they would organize on their own for more and better treatment, and the likelihood that very many state officials would take them seriously if they did, is so small as to be unthinkable."[18] I could see why Sue raged at this author decades later.

Through an internship during college, Sue met Frank Guzman, who brought her to visit a homeless shelter for the first time. Guzman also worked with the Minnesota AIDS Project on the Main Line—the first needle exchange in Minneapolis, named after Bill Main—where she met and became acquainted with others working on the forefront of harm reduction and HIV education not only in Minnesota but nationwide.[19] One of those Minnesota people, Toni St. Pierre, a registered nurse, became a new friend and colleague of Sue's.[20] Sue and Toni discovered that they shared progressive ideas about the importance of needle exchanges and access to harm-reduction services, and wanted to do more for people they observed having a harder time accessing services, and they began reaching out to people in other places, such as the Chicago Recovery Alliance.[21]

They soon decided to focus on the women whom they had witnessed not getting the same access to clean needles and other resources as those available to men, particularly gay men at risk for contracting HIV. Since they both had experiences working with women in crisis, they came up with an idea to create a new model for needle exchange, one that had a focused emphasis on women but did not exclude men. What would harm reduction look like for women drug users who might be too afraid to leave their homes, their children, or their abusive partners? What about women sex workers who were only just being acknowledged as having particular vulnerability to HIV? What if Sue and Toni truly "met them where they were" in the literal sense, as in delivering clean needles to their homes? Meeting people "where they are at" is a commonly used shortcut to explain harm reduction:

meet them exactly where they are, for who they are, right then, and without judgment, which includes accepting their choice to use drugs while offering safer ways to do it. Most importantly, it means seeing their humanity first.

With what I learned quickly to be Sue's signature wit, they named the organization "Women with a Point!," with the exclamation point intended to represent both a needle and an exclamation, just as the name itself had two meanings. When she explained it to me, she smiled broadly and said, "I would say to people, Women with a Point!—we have a point to make and a point to give." Women with a Point! (WAP) incorporated in September 1996 and started the process of becoming a nonprofit. The first funding they received was a small grant from NASEN, the North American Syringe Exchange Network, in order to purchase supplies needed for safe injection kits.[22]

When they founded WAP, Sue and Toni believed that women drug users had unique needs that inspired them not only to do street outreach but to meet women in their homes and apartments. "The way that I've always thought about it, I'm sure generated out of my own life experiences, men were fine in their place. I was never really sure *where* their place was and how [they] fit in. I didn't dislike them. I just thought women needed something more, new." Their idea to focus on women users was a novel approach in needle exchange and harm reduction, and although the Minnesota AIDS Project had a portable needle exchange that operated out of a van, WAP started by going directly to their clients. At first they worked out of their homes assembling outreach bags full of clean syringes, and then hit the streets, particularly Currie Avenue in Minneapolis. Since Sue was working at the time for Branch 3, a Catholic Charities day shelter on East Seventeenth Street where people gathered who used the night shelters on Currie Avenue, she was recognized and known by people who would benefit from her new needle exchange program. She filled up a gym bag with the outreach kits—"syringes, cottons and cookers, condoms, granola bars, socks"—and kept a sharps container at the bottom of the bag to collect used needles. Sue was definitely aware of her create-as-you-go model for WAP, and though she had support from colleagues on both the East Coast and West Coast, they weren't "in the holy land of treatment," the term she and others often used to describe the predominance of the Minnesota Model in Minnesota. Besides word spreading about their syringe exchange services, it was through a grant from the Minnesota Department of Public Health that they were able to rent a small brick storefront on Fifteenth Street, between Nicollet and LaSalle in the Loring Park neighborhood just south of downtown Minneapolis.

The move to the storefront changed many things for WAP. Toni St. Pierre had since moved on to other work, and Sue started applying for larger grants, including one from the CDC for $750,000 to expand the kinds of services they offered.[23] Initially, she and the board were unsure about whether to apply for the grant, but when she called the project officer in charge, they were encouraged to apply. It was a huge application that she undertook with the WAP board chair Gayle Thomas and David Hamilton, a new employee of WAP. They decided to do it for the experience and had no expectations. Sometime later, she got a call from the project officer. "I was on my way to the theater with a friend, and I remember I almost drove off the road. They'd funded us. They had funded us! We went from year one, probably a ten thousand [dollar] budget, to within four years, we are at $750,000. It was huge." They were able to hire more staff, expand their programming, and increase the size of their work space. "We did testing in the jails and in drug court and provided prevention education in prisons," she explained, and she added, they provided "comprehensive harm reduction in a way that doesn't happen ever again here."

Sue's development and grants approach was to be completely forthright to funders about what she wanted to do with the grant money before she ever applied. For a Women's Foundation grant in which she planned to create a women drug user's support group, she recalled explaining to them, "'I want to create a financial planning education for drug-using women.' . . . I said, 'You've got to tell me right now, if you won't consider this idea, I won't consider applying because I don't want to waste my time.'" The grantor funded the group, and Sue advertised the program as "How to manage your drug habit on a budget." She remembered that even the women in the group would look at her like she was "nuts." She believed that one of the best ways to approach harm reduction for women, to increase their chances of finding stability in their lives, was to help remove the chaos and anxiety that surrounded their drug habit. "It's never supposed to be that conversation." The expected conversation, however, "is about being sober, paying your rent, not buying drugs or even considering it." She knew then, and still knows now, that this was considered blasphemy in the world of drug treatment protocol. The group was not about stopping drug use, but about regaining some little bit of control in their own lives.

Edith Springer's training and harm-reduction philosophies profoundly influenced Sue's work. Among her personal papers related to the history of WAP was a double-sided, photocopied, and highlighted handout of Edith Springer's from 1996, "Worker Stances for Clients Who Use Drugs." Sue's budget workshops were a direct offshoot of the harm-reduction philosophy Springer taught around the United States during the 1990s. Sue had highlighted several parts of the handout, and two of these were especially connected to her workshops and overall approach. "The key for the harm reduction worker is to develop *a relationship* with the participant so that there can be an open discussion about the complex reasons/motivations/and meanings surrounding the behavior. . . . You are not there to 'fix' anybody . . . it is the participant's job to develop strategies and solutions that work for them at their own pace."[24]

This philosophical approach was not even in the same realm as the notion that drug users have to "hit rock bottom" and admit "powerlessness" over their addiction. In my shock about the contrast, I mentioned this to Sue, to which she replied, "It's so punitive. It's so judgmental. . . . It's death. I had been one of those women. For some reason I have a very creative, innovative, survival force in me. To be able to share that with other women has always been my driving force." She described the purpose of the group in more detail. It was about banking and how you can have a habit. "You can pay your rent. You can budget your money. Drug use is not mutually exclusive from organization. Your life is not chaotic. You can plan. You can recognize that this is part of it and it serves a role in your life." These are never the messages to women who use drugs, and she wanted to approach their problems from a more empowering place, not a defeating one. Sue went on, "'It's bad, you're wrong.' Everything about that. 'You're an awful mother. You don't love your children.' How much stigma can you heap on? Then you work at dismantling that and providing another point of view."

She knew how this worked and how women could get to a better place in their lives because she herself had survived such adversity. In a harm-reduction model of care, if a social worker doesn't understand that, the chances of the client trusting them, much less stopping or decreasing use, was unlikely. Springer opened a 1991 harm-reduction article about effective AIDS prevention among active drug users with this: "People need to feel worthwhile and empowered in order to make difficult changes in their lives; starting from the perspective that what one does is bad—or that one's entire life is pathological—is a setup for failure."[25]

WAP sponsored a variety of other workshops, all designed to empower and educate its clients on a range of issues. They ran the gamut of "know your rights, safe disposal, how do you write to your congressperson," and even "voters' rights." The women's users group invited the League of Women Voters to come visit them. Sisters of Carondelet who had the Peace House on Nicollet Avenue and who had protested at the School of the Americas in the 1980s and 1990s visited WAP and volunteered their services. To add interest and color to the space, Sue bought "two hundred dollars' worth of posters" from Northern Sun, a 1970s-era political print shop in Minneapolis, and created a collage of posters on the walls of their space.[26] Those posters became conversation starters on human rights, history, and politics among clients. "It was such a wonderful opportunity to educate and open a mind, to put forth other ideas."[27]

When I finally asked Sue how she met her late husband Dave Purchase, she laughed and said slyly, "Everyone knew Dave Purchase." I persisted. "But how did you meet him?" It was 1996, and she was just getting started with WAP. She went to Oakland, California, to attend the first harm-reduction conference held in the United States. "I thought he was a showboat. . . . Dave was a presence. I thought he was a little too full of himself." Maybe he had a reason for being this way, I thought, considering that she was at a conference he organized, by a national organization he founded, after running and founding the first needle exchange in the United States in Tacoma, Washington.[28] He seemed like a big deal to me, actually, considering the radical outreach work he was doing at the time. She demurred, sort of. "Dave was instrumental in starting all the New York programs. He worked throughout the country. He worked throughout the world, programs in Hawaii and Vietnam and Puerto Rico, everywhere. He's this larger-than-life figure. I think he's arrogant and annoying. I have to do business with him."

A year passed, and Sue applied for money from his organization to start the mobile syringe access program that would become WAP. No other places she knew of provided start-up funds for needle exchanges other than NASEN, which meant she had to contact Dave Purchase. She didn't get the grant. "I remember calling him on the phone and saying, 'What's the deal? Where's my money? Why didn't I get some?' Out of that he sent me a little money for needle exchange." A year after that, she was at a drug policy conference in New Orleans when she saw Dave Purchase at a bar, surrounded by conference attendees. She initially planned to avoid him, but later joined the group. "Dave used to hold court in the bar, everybody was there. This was harm reduction in the United States. All these people who are the old timers now were young, having a conversation with him in the bar. It was a good conversation; it was an interesting conversation. He wasn't annoying. It was enjoyable. Then there was an attraction."

In 1998, Sue went to the International Harm Reduction conference in Brazil and met an Australian named Peter Goldsworthy from Sydney. He worked with a company called ASP Plastics. They had recently begun to manufacture and market a personal sharps disposal container for syringes, originally designed by injection drug users (IDUs). They named it Fitpack.[29] The black oval container was a little bigger than a sunglasses case and held ten clean syringes on one side and had a disposal area on the other that could not be opened once the used needles were deposited inside. When full, the whole thing could be safely discarded.

A year after meeting them at the conference, and after the state had created the Minnesota Syringe Access Initiative, Sue wrote a grant with the Minnesota Department of Health to assist with the initiative at WAP. They would educate people about the new law and distribute Fitpack containers. They titled the project "Better Safe than Sorry Disposal Proposal." Based on the successful Australian project model, Pharmacy Fitpack Scheme, they reached out to work with four local pharmacies in Twin Cities neighborhoods known for IV drug use: Uptown and North Side Minneapolis, and the East Side and West Side of St. Paul.[30] The grant allowed them to distribute the Fitpacks that were filled with ten clean needles and syringes, an informational sticker about safe use practices, and a survey card for the research component of the project. People who participated in the research questionnaire at the storefront would also receive a T-shirt that read "Be Blood Aware. Better Safe Than Sorry."

Through this program grant, they gained insights into something they had not really expected, especially given the HIV/AIDS crisis and heightened awareness of transmission, and that was how pharmacies were actually preventing drug users from access to clean, affordable syringes. By this time, the law allowed anyone to buy a ten-pack, but much of the pricing reflected the discretion of the pharmacist based on who was wanting to buy them. Now that she knew the wholesale price of syringes, she could track who was charging more. She remembered a ten-pack being seventy cents wholesale, and drug users were being charged five dollars. "If you were a diabetic, I think it was three dollars. There was a price break. That was interesting, [but] not a surprise." One Minneapolis pharmacy asked for identification and limited the number of visits that a person could have to a pharmacy. The goal of the grant project was "to help alleviate those glitches, get more uniform policies throughout pharmacies, and give access to people, [and] address safe disposal.

For a time, the Fitpack project brought a level of safety to the streets that law enforcement appreciated as well. According to Purchase, the cops didn't have to worry about accidentally getting pricked by a used needle when they went to pat someone down, and it also made it safer for users to return their needles. Since it was difficult to get used needles out of a Fitpack, being prosecuted for drug residue was much less likely. According to Sue, "it was a win-win situation" and a project that really raised awareness among many different groups.

Women with a Point! changed its name to Access Works in early 2000. Though they had always been serving both women and men, in order to expand the scope of their services and clientele, the name change seemed important at the time, and certainly more inclusive. Reflecting on that decision twenty years later, Sue admitted she had regrets about the name change and felt she "caved to public opinion," because she still wanted the focus to be on women's needs, including those who identify as women. She didn't mind helping male clients and knew they had important issues, but she wanted the primary focus to be on women. This outlook reminded me of Planned Parenthood in the same era—men could always access services, but they were not the central part of the organization's mission. The innovative aspect of her focus struck a chord with me—she had an understanding of the impact of trauma on women's lives and saw valid reasons why they needed to be cared for in a trauma-informed way, long before that term was de rigueur in social services. Both her life experiences and her volunteer work related to domestic violence combined seamlessly with the philosophy of harm reduction for drug users. How could that model be incorporated into what she knew would be "trauma-likely" situations? What safe space could she provide for women to seek care and safety, if even just momentarily? Despite the name change, she continued working on behalf of some of society's most marginalized people, locally and nationally.

By her early twenties, Deb Holman had discovered that she was more attracted to women than men and recognized, in retrospect, that many of her "relapse crises" happened because of break-ups with girl-friends. Keeping a job and a "home base" was important to her, and even though she had her share of crises, she knew how to remain employed. She also worked too much, another example of what she referred to as being part of her addictive personality. "I was always a workaholic. So anytime I wasn't using I was working two jobs or three jobs. I definitely still have that issue, too. I have two jobs, and I have for like ten years. I don't know if that's a good thing or a bad thing." She had worked in factories in Cloquet and had a long stint at a photography store in Minneapolis, but most of her work has been in emotionally and physically intense fields. While living in the Twin Cities and going to college at St. Catherine's, one of her first jobs was street outreach with homeless youth through a coordinated program called StreetWorks. Founded in 1994, StreetWorks was a collaborative effort between partner agencies that helped homeless and runaway youth.[31]

The Weedweevils continued to weave in and out of each other's lives and even saved each other's lives. At some point in late April or early May 2002, Deb and Lisa, the childhood friend who had traveled with Sue after high school, went to visit Lisa's brother Joel, the big brother who had christened them the Weedweevils all those years ago. He had recently divorced and was not doing well. He and Deb had dated at one point back in high school, but now she was scared of him. He had rifles and talked about homosexuals. They did go out to a movie—*Blow*, she noted, ironically. She remembered that "they had a good talk."

Two weeks later, after Deb and Lisa had returned home, Joel died by suicide. Deb was sober at the time, "really trying hard to stay on track," and remembered that she managed to get through the entire funeral and gathering afterward in the local hangout, the Rendezvous Bar in Cloquet, where she stayed sober despite the drinking and drug use around her. She drove back to the Twin Cities the next day, palms sweating, just knowing she was going to use. She had been struggling before the funeral, but afterward, it was all just too much.

She got drugs from her neighbor and then proceeded to go on "a four-day bender" with speedballs, a mixture of heroin and cocaine. Deb had been in touch with Sue regularly, since she had been working at Seton Hall and helping with Access Works occasionally. Sue knew Deb was struggling. "I had been communicating with Sue because she's in the 'Goddammit Debbie' mood, the 'Here goes Debbie again.' I've done some crazy things. . . . Apparently, I was going to go to the employee assistance program or something on Monday, whatever day it was. We were supposed to do something together that morning and she hadn't heard from me." That is when Sue went to her house. "She came over and pounded on my door, no answer. I think she was getting ready to leave, and then the neighbor came out and said, 'Deb's fine. She's sleeping on the couch.' Well, I wasn't. Sue said I was shallow breathing, turning blue." Sue got into the apartment, checked Debbie's breathing, and called an ambulance. They administered Narcan, and she was revived.

The overdose was a turning point. She was in the hospital for nine days recovering and trying to convince the doctors that she was not suicidal. She lost her jobs in outreach, was banned from coming near them, and felt that many people had turned their backs on her. What she realized, though, was the danger she had put her life in when she used hard drugs. "At that point I—inside of myself—woke up to how I used drugs. I'm like, 'No, I was not suicidal, but it's suicidal.'" She did agree to go to treatment again, for work-related purposes, hoping to get her job back. Deb made me chuckle at the end of this harrowing story, though, when she smiled and said, "That time I went to Pride Institute. I thought, 'I'll try the gay one this time, see how that goes.'" The Pride Institute, located in Eden Prairie, Minnesota, opened in 1986 to provide residential and outpatient treatment specifically for the LGBTQ+ population, and even though other programs since then marketed being "LGBTQ affirming," the *Alcoholism & Drug Abuse Weekly* noted in 2012 that the Pride Institute continued to be an innovator in its exclusive focus on LGBTQ+ clientele.[32] This was her last time in an inpatient program.

Even though Deb completed treatment, she was fired her from her position, which she understood. Although she was depressed by this, she kept looking for her work anchor, the thing that kept her focused.

She found an outreach position at Simpson Housing, a housing services organization that began in 1982 as an emergency overnight shelter. More than fifteen years later, at the annual May Day parade and festival in Minneapolis, Deb and Sue ran into Deb's former boss at Simpson Housing, Monica Nilssen. They greeted each other, and Deb remembered looking at Sue and saying to them both, "The person who saved my life and the one that gave me a second chance." She asked Monica, "When you hired me did you know I had had this incident?" Monica nodded. Then Deb announced, "Group hug!"

Deb has stayed away from hard drugs ever since the 2002 overdose. She wasn't even aware of how long ago it had been when we spoke. "It's not that I don't get triggered, I just know where I go and what stops me. I'm that person who needs some kind of security, and I don't want to lose it. I am very grateful that I made it through the last one." She believes that owning a home and knowing a lot of people in Duluth has been part of what keeps her on track. That, and working for two street-based outreach organizations. After the overdose, "I just worked . . . got into homelessness. Outreach was my thing. I've always poured my heart into it. I don't have kids, I don't have a family I've got to go home for. I've always been pretty available."

Sue and Dave got married in 1999, and by 2004 their commuter marriage was getting hard to maintain. She had promised Dave she would move to Tacoma at some point, since that was where his work life was based. Sue resigned from Access Works in the fall, and the assistant director, David Hamilton, replaced her as executive director. Sue started working for ASP Plastics, the Australian company that sold the Fitpack. Now settled in Tacoma, she had plenty of harm-reduction opportunities, not only related to the Fitpack job, but with the organizations and conferences that Dave and NASEN organized. She may have been burned out in Minneapolis, but she continued the work of harm reduction nonetheless.

Once she acclimated to Dave's needle exchange program, Sue realized that she had been running a much more comprehensive service back in Minneapolis. Shocked by how much worse things were in Tacoma for stigmatized people on the fringes, she started bending and breaking the "rules." The Tacoma Needle Exchange had a strict one-for-one policy, meaning that participants had to bring in one used needle to get one clean needle. Sue thought that the policy had emerged when Dave was "being glib with *People* magazine during an interview," back in the late 1980s when he first began getting press coverage for his card-table-on-a-street-corner needle exchange.[33] She imagined that's how it became ensconced in the rules of the program he ran. She bristled at this idea, and soon began doing her own thing when she was working at the fixed site exchange van on Fourteenth and G Street in Tacoma. Sometimes people would dig around in the dirt to find a used needle, or would scavenge anywhere to find pieces of syringes or plungers to bring in. "They had to find evidence of a syringe and bring it. Dave had people working for him that were very obedient, but that wasn't me. I was a game changer at the exchange. They'd come on Fridays, and I'd say, 'Five can get you ten.' It wasn't going to be a strict one for one. I wasn't going to be stupid about it, but it wasn't a policy I could abide by." The stories she recalled from this time in her life were as vivid as any other, and her tenacious opinions remained unchanged as well, whether married to the founder of U.S. needle exchanges or not.

One heartbreaking story involved a woman named Linda. Sue began the story as if citing bullet points in a presentation, but the power of each one was hard to absorb before she listed the next one. "This is a story about stigma. Linda had lived on the streets for fifteen years in Tacoma. She was beautiful when she was young. She was from Montana. She had kids that she was estranged from. She did sex work to survive. She had a seizure disorder." Sometimes during our interviews, usually at times just like this one, I struggled to keep up. If listening to these stories was hard, experiencing them firsthand had to have been excruciating. And the telling again, after all these years, had to be difficult for her. Sue persisted while I nodded, took it all in, thankful for the recording device.

She continued. When they first met, Sue helped Linda by keeping her seizure medication secure. People on the streets who didn't need it would steal the pills from her to get high. Linda would come by every day to get her pill. One day she stopped coming. At some point, Linda's friend Troy came by to say that Linda had cancer and had finally been housed due to her terminal illness. Troy said Linda hoped to see Sue before she died. "I finally go to visit Linda. Her belly is really distended, she had liver cancer. Linda had been living with AIDS for twenty years." Sue began checking on her regularly to make sure she had her medications. Linda loved to smoke cigarettes and she loved to smoke crack. "I knew she smoked crack. I'm like, 'Here's the deal. I don't care.' We became very close and I ended up helping her, with the help of Joe the nurse and Linda's boyfriend, we helped her die at home." For Sue, this story in particular was "representative of the stigma, the lack of services, and the lack of caring for people who were homeless, strung out, drug users in Tacoma."

Sue became disillusioned about the impact a basic, one-for-one needle exchange could have on people suffering from multiple oppressions and barriers to care. Given her history, I was not surprised to learn that if a partner she loved and respected didn't honor the fierceness of her commitment to women in these kinds of vulnerable situations, their relationship was likely doomed. I sensed that some part of what Dave had not done was to adequately acknowledge the holes in the system that let women and others fatally fall through. She held him to a higher standard, one on par with her own high standard, and was disappointed when he didn't the make changes she thought were necessary to grow a holistic, surround-care, kind of program. A needle exchange by itself was not adequate. "Needle exchange is a strategy that reduces harm, but it does not mean that it's done with compassion or with any sort of insights or care. It simply exchanges a syringe on a good day." In her view, "The idea behind needle exchange is it builds a bridge to other services." In Sue's thinking about harm-reduction practices, a clean needle should not be all one gets. Despite their differences about harm-reduction philosophies and the dissolution of their marriage, she remained nostalgic about Dave Purchase. "What a human being—certainly human! We had an amazing relationship for about nine years, traveled, worked together, my confidante, his confidante."[34] Sue and Dave split up in 2007, and she moved back to Minneapolis, where she found Access Works still running but much changed.

Rae Eden Frank had worked with Sue on many different projects beginning in 2000. When Sue left for Tacoma, Rae worked with the new executive director David Hamilton, and when he moved on to another job in 2003, she interviewed for and was offered the executive director position for Access Works. Her experience as a former drug user and her empathy for women clients in particular made her a valuable asset. She wrote grants and developed new programs that provided wound care, partnered with neighborhood health clinics, tested for hepatitis C and HIV, increased Narcan distribution, and spearheaded "bad dope" alerts. By 2007, she was worn out. When she learned Sue was coming back to Minneapolis, Rae called to see if Sue wanted to run the organization again. She agreed to step back in temporarily. As a mother of two young daughters, Rae wanted a job less centered on direct services and programming; she found one as executive director of Sobriety High Foundation, a nonprofit that ran four sober high schools in the metro area.

When Sue returned temporarily to Access Works, she noticed that the drug scene had changed in Minnesota. The opioid pain pill crisis was now ten years in, and along with it had come an increase in heroin use and availability. "I was shocked by what had happened there, what had changed. . . . Pills are plentiful. People are coming through the door. . . . They're younger, they're from the suburbs, and they don't look like they belong there. They are there looking to hook up." She stayed for some months at the helm again but realized she didn't "have the magic to save the organization." She was beyond burned out by this point and had experienced loss after loss. "I'm fried. In my own life at the time I had friends dying of cancer. My mother had died, and suicides among other friends, countless overdose deaths in Tacoma. . . . I'd gotten a divorce. People continued to tell me one sad story after another. . . . I couldn't be there anymore." A new director was hired but was only there for a short time before Access Works shut down permanently in 2009. As Rae explained it, "The closing of Access Works was a casualty of the 2008 recession. Donations and grants from small family foundations dried up. A lot of nonprofits in the Twin Cities closed, downsized, or merged between 2007 and 2009."[35]

Sue stayed in Minneapolis for a few years after this, started a graduate school program, and worked at Simpson Housing where she helped organize a new harm-reduction-based housing program for women with chronic homelessness and substance issues. She liked the work, but she was still struggling with grief and anxiety—more close friends and family had passed away. In 2013, she packed up her car, visited friends around the country, and then moved to Colorado to spend time in the mountains and be near her daughter. This was where she was living when we met over the phone in early April 2017.

When Sue came back to Minnesota that May to see family and attend the White Earth Nation's Sixth Annual Harm Reduction Summit, she encouraged me to meet her there. Held over three days at the Shooting Star Casino and Event Center in Mahnomen, Minnesota, the summit had grown since its origins and now attracted people from all over the United States. The world of harm reduction is vast, vibrant, and multifaceted, and the attendees mirrored this fact. The themes of the conference that year included "Decolonization, Sovereignty and Health Justice," "Self-Care" for people working in substance abuse, health care, and related fields, and "Exploring New Partnerships" to improve access to care. Public health professionals, social workers, physicians, nurses, activists, and advocates of all kinds filled the conference rooms. I attended an emotionally stirring panel that featured testimonials from young mothers who were participants in MOMS (Maternal Outreach and Mitigation Services), a supportive, culture-centered, White Earth treatment program. I listened while a nervous young public health epidemiologist presented what he called "Indian Country" overdose data, only to find himself being questioned intensely about the "cause of death" details in his data by Indigenous elder mothers who wanted better answers from state officials. They were certain that some of the deaths he was claiming as suicides were not in fact suicides but overdoses. It was a powerful moment to witness. At another session, a San Francisco–based harm-reduction expert offered a workshop about how to build trust among needle exchange participants in order to teach safer injection strategies. The innovative dedication of conference participants was impressive on its own, but the White Earth Nation organizers, whose experiences at ground zero for opioid overdose deaths—seven times that of whites in Minnesota—made the event a painful combination of hope and crisis. I was incredibly grateful to attend and devastated to realize how much more work had to be done.[36]

Back in Minneapolis that next week, Sue introduced me to her dear pal Deb Holman and we made a plan to meet up. Samantha Aamot and Sara Ludewig, my two steadfast student research assistants, and I drove to Duluth to meet her and several others working in social services related to housing and substance use, among others. Deb suggested a café north of downtown with a close-up view of Lake Superior, and even though it was windy and a bit chilly, we sat at a patio table near the street. She wanted to be able to smoke. No matter what time of the year I visit, Duluth is always windy and chilly, especially downtown near the vast expanse of Lake Superior. Deb tells me she loves this weather and even commented that if it were any warmer than this (it was barely above 50 degrees Fahrenheit) she'd be too hot. I smiled bravely and tried to settle in for our brisk chat. As we talked, she waved to several people she knew, and they waved back. Once, she interrupted her own story, to say, "Cops . . . Oh, I like him," and waved as a City of Duluth Police SUV drove slowly past us. She mentioned that some people are critical of her positive relationship with local police, citing issues of police mistreatment and aggression. She believes strongly in police accountability for excessive force, but in her outreach work, she wanted to model something else. "I try to portray good interactions with the police because I do interact with them in a good way quite often. They're very helpful to me, and I want people to see that. It helps the homeless cause I think, too."

Located where we were, even for just over an hour, I could easily see that much of her work was built on these relationships, even if she and the police officers sometimes disagreed about the best way to solve a problem. Of her street-based clients, she confirmed that, too, was built on recognition and trust. "You just gotta build the relationships and get people to trust you. . . . I always like having that face-to-face contact. You've got to. Then you know who they are." Working with a variety of different agencies at a time seemed natural to her, and having people see it in action was essential.

Duluth, with its population of eighty-five thousand and the second largest University of Minnesota campus, has a history of creating formal and informal affiliations between organizations to coordinate community services more efficiently and humanely. Greg Anderson, the social service supervisor for St. Louis County Public Health Human Services, works in Chemical Dependency Services for the county and agreed to meet with me. He joked that this history of collaboration must be because of "something in the drinking water." Joking aside, he elaborated:

It's something that I witnessed when I first came to the community in 1987, and there is just something here that is just part of the culture and the value of being able to work together and support each other even though we may not agree on other various items or values in life. When we have a common purpose or see a problem that needs to be solved, we can push our differences aside to work jointly and in a collaborative fashion.[37]

One example he gave was the New San Marco, a residential supportive housing for chronic alcoholics that allowed fifty residents to continue to use alcohol while also providing case management, linking them to primary care services, and offering access to treatment should they choose it.[38] They discovered that when fixed housing was provided, residents decreased their alcohol use and some sought treatment for it.

Another was OARS, the Opioid Abuse Response Strategies group, set up in 2012 and comprised of the Duluth Department of Health, a police officer representative, a pharmacy professor from the university, medical professionals, treatment directors, and other outreach workers, including Deb, who attended occasionally. In a quintessentially Minnesota fashion, Greg described the transition from pain pills to heroin so neutrally that I almost missed that he was talking about drug dealers.

> When [pills] were no longer easily accessed, the entrepreneurship of others—reflecting back on supply and demand—basically said, "[if] they can't have prescription medications, we have something that will fit their need and we will be able to provide it at a price that will be good for us and affordable for them." That started to swing or shift into heroin.

Minnesotans might be teased for this kind of passive, neutral phrasing, but in the context of an opioid epidemic and especially when discussing the philosophy of harm reduction, his approach was as refreshing as Sue and Deb's. It was also kind. He held no malice; he just wanted people he is paid to serve to get the help they need. Of human services work as a whole, he said everyone in the field must understand addiction and drug use.

> It doesn't matter if you're doing child protection or working with the elderly: chemical dependency and addiction is going to be part of your work. One of the things we are working on from a department standpoint through our Substance Abuse Prevention Intervention Initiative is attempting to put substance use disorder training as a core training function for new social workers, new employees coming into the department. We're not there yet, but we're getting much closer.

Despite these efforts, Deb remains frustrated by what usually causes gaps in services—whether it is a lack of funding and shelter space or not, some people fall through the cracks because of long-standing rules and idiosyncrasies guiding governmental and nonprofit bureaucracies. "There's some things about the shelter that are totally punitive that drive me crazy. . . . I can argue a lot, and I do advocate a lot, to the point where my boss says, 'You're a pain in the ass.'" She agreed. "That's my job!" Yet she does appreciate the leadership efforts that Duluth social service organizations and agencies have made to coordinate care among themselves on behalf of clients. If a client tells the emergency room nurse one problem and the detox center another, "now we can all coordinate" at regular meetings to provide the best assistance possible.

When I asked about what kinds of drug use she was seeing on the streets, she pointed out what is probably obvious: people with chronic alcohol dependency are the ones most visible on the streets in Duluth. Illegal drug use usually causes people to hide out. She noted that outreach to opioid users has been difficult, but she was nevertheless trying to figure out a way to get Narcan into the hands of as many of those users as possible. It was challenging to find them, though. "I know a good number of people that are using heroin but they're not like camping out in a tent. They're hiding out in a drug house. Some of them are in tents, I guess. They tend to not come around. . . . If you're homeless and using heroin you're underground."

Deb keeps her eye out for everyone who needs help, their pets included. "Somehow, I started taking pets home. . . . I fostered a ton of dogs." They have accumulated in her home and her heart over a number of years. The first foster dog experience was during the winter of 2005. "This homeless guy had him in his backpack. He was just this beautiful little puppy. It was like twenty below, and he's drunk. Bless his heart." Pets are not allowed in shelters, and sometimes these pets inevitably became hers because their owners never returned for them or even died. "Benny and Joy, a couple, were out here. I asked if I could take the dog home. The rest is history. I think Benny's eleven now. The real Benny died." Her current tableaux of five different dogs appears regularly on her social media pages. One summer she posted photos of a vandalized encampment in the woods near Duluth in hopes of soliciting donations of new tents, sleeping bags, and clothes. Even though she does get a lot of donations when she asks for supplies on Facebook, she noted the discrepancy between the number of "likes" she gets for her menagerie of dogs versus the "likes" for the people who need shelter. She shrugged it off, though. "Yeah, I think it's funny people like my dog pictures more." Her use of the word "funny" struck me as quintessentially Minnesotan, a sharp yet indirect critique, couched in such a benign word.

Since 2005, Deb has kept what she calls "the Duluth list" of unhoused people who die every year in the city. She has been the person who reads it every year as part of a statewide memorial ceremony. She remains very committed to this annual ritual, and even joked that she was told by the organizers that she can continue doing so "until my name is on the list!" Her compassion and empathy has to be balanced by something light, even if it is a bit dark. Just like the ongoing and increasing numbers of overdose deaths in the state, dying while living without shelter is another problem that seems far from being solved. In July 2020, the number of people who had died was already at forty. Deb's Facebook page has also served as an informal memorial site, too. Interspersed with her dogs and news articles are photos of the deceased and kind rest-in-peace messages about them from her. Recently, she felt she needed to clear something up for her "friends."

> FYI/
> When I post that people have passed away a lot of folks say "Sorry Deb." It's a community loss. It's not something I do for personal sympathy. Each life deserves and needs to be remembered. Some I know well and some I don't. Each loss is sad and often tragic.
> I definitely go to too many funerals.
> I want to explain the reason I do it. Seems like a good time.
> Every year there is a state wide memorial honoring those who died while homeless or may have been homeless at some point in their life. . . .
> Many have no obituary or funeral/remembrance
> For 2020 we already have 40 names, 40 people to remember. That's too many.
> But we will remember & honor all of them.[39]

In 2019, Deb convinced her friend Sue that there was a lot of work to be done in northern Minnesota. Sue was ready for a move and decided to see if she would like living on home turf again. As we sat down for a third interview, and in her typical poetic fashion, she noted, "I arrived back around the 11th of July, 2019. . . . I had left northern Minnesota when I was nineteen years old on the 15th of July 1979. So, the forty-year road trip had come to an end! Right? It had come to an end."[40] We were sitting in her high-ceilinged apartment in an older brick, rowhouse-style building in view of Lake Superior. Sue spends her free time now at a park overlooking the lake that is full of rose gardens, a Works Progress Administration–era flagstone amphitheater, benches, and trails.

Sue reconnected with harm-reduction friends, worked for the Rural AIDS Action Network, and in less than a year started her own nonprofit organization, Harm Reduction Sisters. She is back at work distributing not only safe injection kits and Narcan kits, but also wound care kits, fentanyl test strips, and sharps containers; she also collects syringes for safe disposal. She does this by car, accepting calls and texts from participants at least five days a week. She has received grants from some of the organizations she used to work with, including NASEN and the Comer Foundation. In the first year alone, Harm Reduction Sisters distributed over five hundred thousand syringes and well over four thousand doses of Narcan. When my eyes nearly popped out of my head, she nodded and said, "Yeah, Debbie and her suggestion that mobile was needed and necessary up here, she was spot on about that!"

The geographic area she serves is enormous, rural, and isolated, even more so once COVID-19 arrived in March 2020. She listed a dozen towns in three counties and two reservations, as well as Superior, Wisconsin, Duluth's neighboring city to the east. She serves clients on the Fond du Lac Reservation and arranges meeting points for people who are then distributing the supplies to even more remote areas. No one-for-one exchange has meant that demand is probably higher for her, but she doesn't mind. The other syringe exchange in Duluth is a store front and follows the Dave Purchase model. She is trying to change the drug-using culture in Northern Minnesota by insisting on clean syringes for each use. Sue was surprised by the different kinds of drugs being injected, besides methamphetamine and heroin, and really concerned about HIV and hepatitis C transmission, which she noticed very few people talk about. She wants to educate people on the best safe use practices. "It just blows my mind. The standard, the culture up here is to reuse syringes time after time after time for months on end. Not only are you going to reuse them and you're going to sharpen them on a matchbook, you're going to share them with your friends!" The recent HIV outbreak in St. Louis county, where Duluth is located, has proven that her concerns about the consequences of reusing needles were on the mark. In a county that typically sees one to five cases per year since late 2019, they have since confirmed thirteen new cases as of April 2021.[41]

Besides trying to fill public health education gaps for drug users, Sue has other ideas for Harm Reduction Sisters in the near future. She wants to develop an art studio and name it "the Art of Harm Reduction, to have a place where people can do art, whether it is painting or spoken word—a creative outlet that helps people manage their trauma, their symptoms, their drug use, that provides a safe place where people can explore who they are with drugs, or without them." She also wants to start a writing group for women called Women of Substance and has been encouraged by the positive response about the idea from artists and writers she's met since returning home. "I think once people have an opportunity to do something different, are introduced to another way of thinking, it's life changing. Just like it was for me. Really, that is my goal. I've come full circle."

CHAPTER 5

Dissecting Stigma
Treatment Reimagined

In midsummer 2014, my daughter Madeleine and her boyfriend Brandon went to inpatient treatment in two different places simultaneously. We could never be sure, but we held out hope that this would be the last time. Every week our family visited them on different days and times, traversing the metro area from the western suburbs of Minneapolis to St. Paul's Midway neighborhood. The contrast between the two institutions could not have been more extreme. My daughter was at an internationally esteemed, suburban facility on a multiacre campus. Full of floor-to-ceiling windows, carpeting, comfy furniture, and contemplative gardens, the place exuded healing and introspective solitude. A large basketball court, nature paths, benches, and flower-drenched trellises dotted the large outdoor spaces adjacent to the building. At the other institutional extreme, her boyfriend was at a bare-bones, scrappy-looking treatment center in an old brick building on a major St. Paul thoroughfare. While her visiting hour could be held outside in manicured gardens, his weekly visits occurred in a windowless, basement dining room that smelled of ketchup and bleach, where everyone sat in uncomfortably close proximity to other visiting families' personal conversations. A picnic table, a tree, and a small concrete pad comprised the entirety of his outdoor options. The place felt quasi-institutional, like a cross between a hospital and an old-style residential flophouse.

Yet over several weeks visiting these two very different spaces, I realized that they offered nearly identical inpatient treatment programming. The only difference was the setting. And money. One was for clients with financial resources or "good" insurance plans, those usually affiliated with corporate and state jobs; the other was for clients with fewer resources, who had lower-benefit plans or were on

state-funded medical insurance.[1] The racial and class differences between the clientele were also obvious. Some treatment centers, like
Hazelden Betty Ford, don't accept medical assistance—they don't have
to in order to keep their business afloat—and, frankly, introducing
Medicaid clients would upset and challenge the more privileged social standing of the organization's current and early history treating
professionals, priests, and celebrities. Generations-long economic in-
equalities and corresponding health disparities meant that access to
comfortable, amenable spaces to recover from addiction was unlikely
for the men in Brandon's treatment center. If the client had been involved in a nonviolent, drug-related crime they might prefer any kind
of space over being in jail. On the one hand, these elitist assumptions
have allowed the stereotype of poor, criminalized drug users to continue to reproduce itself in a revolving-door system of subpar facilities. On the other, many of the men at my son-in-law's rehab were
there by court order; he told me that he steered clear of these guys as
much as possible because they did not all take the services provided
to them as seriously as he did. He worried that their cocky ambivalence could put the success of his own recovery at risk.[2] He embraced
the predominantly Twelve Step–based program but also accepted and
absorbed every innovative program or speaker, in particular Refuge
Recovery, a Buddhist model, and motivational interviewing.[3]

The flexibility that the founders of the Minnesota Model believed
they were incorporating into addiction treatment has had the effect
of making treatment failures, "relapses," part of the chronic nature of
the disease. Rick Moldenhauer, a Minnesota Department of Human
Services consultant, oversees the State Opioid Treatment Authority,
and summarized the tail-chasing, failure-provoking nature of what
happens when the "academically driven" Minnesota Model encounters
generational drug use, trauma, and multiple barriers to well-being:

> With what we [now] know about FASD [fetal alcohol spectrum
> disorder] and neuroplasticity—how things affect the brain and
> how the brain responds to things—to take someone who has
> been an active rip-and-run heroin addict for the last five years
> and assume that they are going to be able to engage in a fairly
> literature-based experience of reading . . . the *Big Book* and com-
> pleting these workbooks on Steps One through Five all in the

span of twenty-eight days . . . those two are incongruous. They don't work well together.

Moldenhauer's insight about what happens next in this situation was all too familiar, as I had heard many stories like it. "An individual client may fall behind, and may not get their assignments done on time, and depending on the sensitivity of the staff, they are seen as resistant to treatment, or not 'surrendering' themselves. They blame the clients. The clients get frustrated and act out. Then they get washed out of the programs."[4]

In a drug-treatment system that is primarily based on an aftercare protocol where individual clients must devote constant mental and spiritual attention to their own recovery—through support groups such as AA—the injustices of a highly racialized, class-based, uneven system of punishments and unsuccessful programming largely remain hidden. The formerly addicted person who relapses in this treatment paradigm conveniently becomes the one to blame. If they failed at sobriety it was, in the final reckoning, a personal problem that they ultimately had control over, despite the acceptance of addiction as a disease. The predominance of and reliance on a powerful combination of long-held moral concepts of individual free will and the familiar yoke of the American bootstrap myth has long hidden the ineptitudes and injustices of the system we call rehab or drug treatment. These two myths, upheld by legal, cultural, medical, and social institutions, have had the effect of making drug addiction primarily the problem of the individual alone, and worse yet, the treatment most people get will likely be based on their race, gender, and access to economic resources.

After interviewing several dozen people over four years, I had hoped to discover that the severity of the opioid epidemic might have goaded the abstinence-only stalwarts to change, might have provoked humane and lasting criminal justice reforms, and that innovative treatment protocols would already be in the process of being thoroughly implemented. After all, we have evidence-based science and medicine for opioid dependence, an ever-expanding knowledge of psychology and neuroscience, and thousands of inpatient and outpatient treatment centers to provide space and services for healing. Even in the midst of a horrible epidemic, I knew I was being overly optimistic.

History teaches us that most significant social changes happen incrementally over a long time, even when there is sustained focus on new ideas, protocols, and policy. In this context, and with our social proclivity as Americans to focus on individualism and ingenuity, I found myself drawn to the stories of people who worked within established treatment systems but who eventually decided to forge their own paths to address problems they couldn't solve within the confines of those systems.

These mental health and addiction service providers took individualism to heart and created models of care that were more intentionally centered on individual clients' needs and wishes for their own treatment outcomes. They paid special attention to the impact of trauma and to cultural and religious differences, and envisoned care that was above all person-centered. Although a robust, nationally coordinated solution to the opioid epidemic has not yet emerged, these three have worked hard to implement positive changes to addiction treatment methods. Whether they worked to change the system from within, created a new model, or focused on targeting a particular need in their community, the professionals featured in this chapter reflect some of the best innovative and adaptive ways that addiction treatment is changing for the better. Julie Hooker, who has a deep understanding of addiction and trauma, created her own treatment center to help people who are among the most stigmatized and traumatized in our society. Paula DeSanto, having worked in mental health institutions and programs, had the audacious vision to create a model she named Minnesota Alternatives in response to a need she saw for options to the Minnesota Model. And Yussuf Shafie, a social worker and Somali immigrant, responded to an unmet need in the East African population for culturally specific addiction and mental health treatment.

Julie Hooker
Resurrection Recovery/Avenues Recovery, St. Paul, Minnesota

The concert hall at the student union was nearly full when I arrived on a cold Friday morning in late January 2017. The University of Minnesota Center for Chemical and Mental Health hosted a two-day workshop with Dr. Gabor Maté, a Canadian physician from Vancouver, British Columbia, who is well known for his trauma-informed analysis about the causes of substance use disorder.[5] I signed up because I had recently read his popular book about addiction, *In the Realm of Hungry Ghosts*, and wanted to hear more. A seat next to me was free, and since bulky coats take up a lot of space during Minnesota winters, I used it for my coat and bag. Just as the program began, a middle-aged woman with a big smile and spiky blond hair asked me if the seat was available. "Of course!" I quickly stuffed my coat and bag under my feet. She settled in, and the speakers were introduced.

Dr. Phyllis Solon was a speaker at the event, and she spent the first session discussing her research on adverse childhood experiences to set the stage for what Maté would build on—that traumatic experiences in childhood can often lead to substance use disorders. She said that "traumatic memory is like phantom limb pain."[6] I knew exactly what she meant. Solon's work dovetailed perfectly with Maté's ideas about addiction. After a lunch break, he took the stage.

Among physicians, Maté's argument about the cause of addiction is controversial, and I understood why, but in the context of his past and the demographics of his patient base, it made sense. He described himself as "a medical doctor in Vancouver's drug ghetto," where he worked at the Portland Hotel Society, a nonprofit that provides housing and medical care for "the nonhousable." As staff physician, he tended the "hard-drug addicts," as he called them—people who experienced neglect, violence, and poverty in their childhoods and then, no surprise, continued on into their adulthood as drug users. His patients suffered mightily from the consequences of long-term addiction, and yet he understood that drugs helped them escape the "hell realm of overwhelming fear, rage, and despair."[7] Maté has a melancholy, wise demeanor that when combined with his humble, self-reflective cadence on stage, made the experience of watching him somewhat mesmerizing. He had some slides but didn't read from them. He spoke contemporaneously about childhood and parenting, attachment and love, the War on Drugs ("a war on human beings"), and the causes of addiction, all while peppering his talk with names of authors, studies, and statistics. The core of his argument: "Not all addictions are rooted in abuse or trauma, but I do believe they can all be traced to painful experience. A hurt is at the center of *all* addictive behaviors."[8] Even though he admitted that viewing addiction as a brain disorder or disease was better than the moral "drug use is a choice" model, he suggested a third approach—one that includes addressing the stresses, fears, and traumas that he believes underlie all forms of addiction.

When he started to tell a story about his own experience with an addiction, the woman next to me and I simultaneously whispered to ourselves: "his classical CD addiction." We smiled at each other in surprise. During the next two breaks that day, I learned that her name was Julie Hooker. We discovered that we knew many people in common, all related to the topic of addiction and the opioid epidemic. I was surprised our paths had not previously crossed and yet was thrilled that they finally did in such a serendipitous way. She told me parts of her own addiction story and shared that she had recently opened her own treatment center. She happily agreed to be interviewed.

A week later, I drove to the offices of Resurrection Recovery, the outpatient treatment center she founded in 2015. It was located on the back side of the Scenic Hills Shopping Center, a tucked-away, yellow and brown brick strip mall on St. Paul's East Side that was also home to a Dollar Store, a panaderia, a law office, a laundromat, and a dental clinic. As soon as I walked in, she jumped right in, telling me about barriers her clients face and how she's working to change the system for them. Her energy and passion for the work she does made the typical formalities associated with beginning oral history interviews completely unnecessary. A few minutes later, I interjected to make sure I got the proper verbal permission, hit record, and let her keep going, not wanting to miss anything she said.

Smiling broadly, Julie described herself as "a native Minnesotan. I'm a blond-haired, blue-eyed Swedish-Norwegian girl, Lutheran, ate lutefisk and lefse at Christmas every year."[9] Her father worked for Community Action Programs, and her mom stayed home to care for Julie and her five siblings. They moved around a lot but mostly stayed in the Twin Cities area. She was quick to say her family upbringing was full of love and affection, very little drama, and no neglect, abuse, or abandonment. There was a lot of alcohol, though, and she started getting sips of beer from her father's cans around age eight or nine. She fondly remembered her dad drinking beer. "He wasn't mean. . . . He was more fun. I'd be like, 'Can I have some money, Dad? Can I get you another beer, Dad?' The reward for going to get him another beer was the first sip out of the can. I had learned that that was a reward for doing something good. . . . I didn't know that that was unusual." At that time in Minnesota, it was legal for a teenager to drink alcohol at a bar if their parent was present and stayed with you. For her high school graduation in 1975, her dad bought a keg of beer for her party. "It wasn't a scary or negative thing when people drank. It was fun and everybody had a good time." Alcohol was never an issue for Julie, but when cocaine arrived on the social scene in the 1980s, she said, "that was a big deal."

In 1978, Julie traveled to Oregon for a vacation and "stayed for twenty-three years." She fell in love with Oregon and then fell in love with her husband. They settled into life in a commune near Harlan, Oregon, halfway between Corvallis and Newport in the coast range. "It was a cool thing to do. I am kind of a hippie at heart." And she wasn't kidding—she played the dulcimer, guitar, and piano, and described herself as an "old Joni Mitchell fan." Although living on the commune remains one of her fondest memories, after two years she and her husband moved into town because she missed "running water and a washing machine, a toaster, and flushing toilets." She tried cocaine for the first time with him, and they grew marijuana plants for their own use, but their use never "got out of hand." For a long time, everything was manageable, and life was good.

After several years of trying unsuccessfully to have children, Julie learned she would need to have surgery to make that possible. Once their first child was born and her focus shifted to mothering, life with her husband became difficult. "There was a lot of betrayal and a lot of abandoning the principles of the vows we took." Her memory is that he had trouble sharing her with their children. After their second daughter was born, they divorced. "That's when things just went kind of south for me." And by south, she meant heroin. The very first man she dated after the divorce was, according to Julie, "a career heroin addict." She tried it almost right away, with just a little hesitation. Quickly, so quickly, "it went from no big deal to oh my gosh now this is a devastating thing. It's really hard to get out of once you're in. I've heard many heroin addicts, and myself included, say, 'The very first time I did it, it was like, where have you been all my life?' That's exactly what happened to me. It just felt wonderful."

Soon after that, she spiraled into selling cocaine and heroin to get more of both, but mostly she needed the heroin. She was bewildered by her own actions, even when she was deep in it. "How did this happen? . . . I'm a mom, I've got these little kids. I worked like hell to be able to have children, and here I am going, 'What the hell is happening to me?'" A few years later, when her daughters were six and eight years old, a SWAT team of police and DEA agents raided her home with guns ready to fire. They used a percussion bomb to shatter her front window, traumatizing her little girls, who were sleeping in their bedroom. Julie was naked, now down on the floor, and one of the men put a gun to her head and his knee in her back, "Don't move!" She started to tear up telling me this, even thirty years later.

> I remember turning my head and seeing my daughter standing in the hallway. Oh my God, it was horrifying. I don't have any violence. I don't have any guns. The kids witness it, and then they try to hand the kids teddy bears. They came in with teddy bears! What the hell is wrong with you? . . . I am handcuffed. They threw a towel over me. I couldn't even hug my kids.

Her boyfriend wasn't there at the time, though he often stayed with her. He got charged with "frequenting," though it was mostly his drug business. Julie was charged with multiple felonies: possession with intent to distribute, child endangerment, and endangering the welfare of a minor, times two.

She was immediately grateful for the joint custody agreement she had with her ex-husband because the girls weren't put into foster care, though they could have been if she hadn't spoken up right then. "I remember one of the officers was saying, 'Take them to child protection services.'"

She said, "No! I've got joint custody. You're calling their dad. Here's his number."

The officer replied, "Isn't he a drug addict, too?"

"You sure didn't do your research."

Her biting, sarcastic comment to the officer made me laugh, even in the middle of such a painful story, but I didn't feel too bad—Julie was laughing, too, still angry and yet also proud of her gumption. That she said it while in handcuffs, covered by a towel, to a SWAT officer astonished me. I learned that putting a little punch of humor into a painful story was a common practice of hers, a wry connection point to lighten things up for a moment. She went right on to make her more important point: "The assumption was there that he must be [an addict], too. I had to fight with them." The officers contacted the girls' father, and they did not to go into child protection. He took the girls right away, but because he and his new wife had two children of their own and were living in subsidized housing that limited the number of people in their home, his family of six ended up living in a shelter until another place could be secured. This still pained her.

Julie was arrested through an informant-controlled buy, and she said that had the agents come the day before they would have found a lot more to charge her with. As it was, they found less than a gram of drugs in her home and she was sentenced to seventy days in jail and sixty months on probation. The child endangerment felony was dropped in a plea deal promise she made to not sell drugs ever again. Releases from county jails usually happen early in the morning, often while it is still dark outside. Julie was given a bus token and told to go see her probation officer, who wouldn't be at work for another four hours. "I'm out at five o'clock in the morning. What am I supposed to do? It's dark. What am I supposed to do?" Naively, I asked her, "You can't go back to your house?" She schooled me.

> I don't have a house. I've been in jail. I lost everything. I lost every-
> thing ten times over. There's a saying, "Go to jail, lose your shit."
> That's just what happens unless somebody had been there to take
> care of all my stuff. It's gone. The landlord came in and took all
> the stuff. I lose it all. You have tons of friends when you have it all
> in place, and the minute you're not there, they're gone. I have no
> place to live, I have no support system in place, I have no money,
> I have no job. I'm not even a mom anymore. I have no responsi-
> bilities. What do I do? I went to the dope house where I knew I
> could find some people that would let me in.

Another time before this one, when she was let out before dawn, she was nervous to walk by herself to an office building and wait in the dark for three hours. So she walked around more familiar places in town for the entire morning. "I was out on what they called 'the stroll.' It was probably noon. A police officer pulled up and went, 'Get in the car.' I hadn't even been out of jail for six hours when I got arrested again for failing to appear with my probation officer." She was never offered any support services in jail. "Nobody came to see me in jail saying, 'What can we do when you get out? How can we help you? What can we do to support you? What are your goals? Can we help you get the kids?'" She tried to figure it all out on her own but admitted that her efforts were weakened because by this point she felt like "a worthless piece of you-know-what. . . . I just screwed everything up. Look what I just did to those kids. Not just in that instance but over years. Look what I just did. It perpetuated everything." She would continue to get arrested, go to jail, and be let out at dawn. The only treatment offered in the county jail then was the opportunity to attend AA meetings. She would go because she'd get out of her cell; it did not help her heroin addiction.

Humiliations continued to pile up, but of course these had no influence on her addiction. Julie interrupted her own chronology to tell me what she called "a funny story" related to being humiliated on a regular basis as a drug user. As things got worse and worse for her, prostitution became a viable option. "I will never forget the first time when I went into court and they call your name and they read the charges . . . 'Julie Hooker, prostitution' and the courtroom erupts in laughter. Even the judge was covering his mouth. My attorney started laughing. . . . This was so humiliating, and you would think, would this not be enough?" The only misdemeanor she ever got was for prostitution—all the others were felonies—but being mocked still stung, regardless of the pun her last name offered the courtroom.

Oregon began drug court around the same time Julie kept being arrested on heroin charges, and since she had no prior anything—not even a parking ticket—she was a good candidate for being remanded to the new program. Yet the care she found in 1990s drug treatment offered very few opportunities for a successful recovery. Humiliating drug users in group sessions and in their day-to-day inpatient living was integral to a treatment model known as Synanon. In 1958, Charles "Chuck" Dederich broke off from his Los Angeles area AA group to create a more powerful and effective peer-led program. He believed that heroin users were more hardened by the consequences of their illegal addiction and its connection to crime. He believed that the nonjudgmental, personal sharing used in AA was too gentle an approach. He developed a group process that relied on confrontation and ridicule to force people to address their moral failings.[10] Similar to what Deb Holman experienced in Minnesota in the 1980s, Julie had to wear a sign that said "Master Manipulator" and stand in the center of the group while everyone took turns describing how manipulative she was. She laughed sarcastically. "Of course, when we are humiliated, we are going to stop the behavior!" If only the cure was so easy.

Julie described how the method tried to tear people down and build them back up, getting rid of the person's ego in order to start again from scratch. "I already felt shame. Ten times what they could give me. [They] don't even know what I felt."

I asked why she never tried methadone during those years she was in and out of jail and treatment. She referred to her past as a heroin dealer and how she perceived methadone clinics at that time. "I was the girl in the parking lot at the methadone clinic. You could come out with your carryouts and I'd trade you a little piece of heroin, and I had the juice lined up in my fridge for backup. . . . That was a joke to me . . . the federal government was your dope dealer." And, for her, the added humiliation of having to stand in line outside a building very early in the morning while people drove by gawking was just too much.[11]

Julie experienced two accidental heroin overdoses, one around 1990 in a stairwell of an apartment building, and the other, the last time she ever used heroin, on December 28, 1996. In both cases she was dumped by her using friends. Before they left her in the stairwell they called an ambulance, and an EMT revived her with Narcan. This first overdose didn't stop her drug use or the associated criminal activity "with a gang of thieves going from town to town boosting from stores and buying heroin, just this terrible life." She felt caught up in a system without a clear way out. She understood why her friends left her. "The fear is we've all got warrants or we're doing criminal activity, we're all going to jail. We can't get caught up in this whole thing." The cycle kept perpetuating itself.

The last overdose, five years later, was a continuation of the same situation. She didn't have her daughters in her life; she was unemployed, still running around with people. They were in a motel room, and when she used that time she remembered thinking, "No, no, no" and feeling that split second "when you can't take it back. I thought I was dead." She woke up on her own twelve hours later on the floor and noticed her ID next to her body. A motel maid was "kind of kicking at me, saying 'You have to pay for another day.'" Her friends left her for dead. They didn't call an ambulance. They left her ID so she would be identified. "Who does that? I had been part of that whole thing for a long time and that day I went, 'I can't.'" She knows that many people call this kind of experience divine intervention. She takes a more pragmatic approach. "I didn't see any bright lights. I didn't hear God talk to me. I didn't have anything like that. I woke up to a motel maid kicking

me telling me I had to pay for another day. That experience trans-
formed me. I got up and gathered myself, and I called the only person
that I knew I could call, my ex-husband. I said, 'Take me to detox.'"

Julie had been to detox so often that she and the staff were on a
first-name basis. In Oregon at the time, a person could stay for ten
days. When she arrived, she pushed the button on the door, announc-
ing, "Hey, it's Julie." The person on the intercom replied, "Hey, honey,
welcome home" and buzzed her in. She convinced the staff to let her
stay well beyond the ten days—probably three weeks or more. She kept
telling them that she couldn't go "out there, out there" again, meaning
back to her drug-using life. "This is what I need. I need to earn an honest day's work. I need to be in a safe surrounding with other people
who are supportive." They told her about a new kind of living situation
that was just being introduced into Oregon, the Oxford House group,
a national organization founded in Silver Spring, Maryland, by Paul
Molloy in 1975, when the sober house he was living in was going to be
closed. He and his housemates, all recovering from alcohol and drugs,
decided they could run a house on their own.[12] A new Oxford House
was opening about thirty miles away from where she had been living
in Salem, Oregon.[13] She interviewed with them and was accepted as a
resident. At that point, she owed two thousand hours of community
service to the state for her drug charges or she would be put in jail
again. She wrote a letter to the judge proposing that she be able to
clock her community service hours for the Oxford House organization instead of "shoveling shit at the zoo or picking up trash on the
freeway." She described herself as being "very manipulative" when she
said to him, "'I want to give back to the community from which I took
so much.' It was all bullshit at the time, truly, but I don't know what
inspired me to do that." I took issue with her description of being manipulative, but she would not back off of that idea. "I look back, and I
wasn't being altruistic and going 'I just really want to help people.' I
wanted to get those hours off my plate."

She jumped into the Oxford House movement full time. Oxford
Houses are democratic, self-run, and self-supporting single-sex resi-
dences for people in recovery from alcohol and drug addiction. Residents pay rent and share all housekeeping responsibilities. Abstinence
is required, and if someone uses, they have to leave. They may appeal
to be voted back in by the rest of the residents, and plenty are. They
hold house meetings, conduct business meetings, and generally just

look out for each other. Julie reveled in the democratic and communal nature of the organization. It fit her personality to live communally, and she thrived being responsible for her part in the house without an authority figure telling her what to do. Shortly after she moved in, she was shocked when the other residents voted her in as the treasurer for the house, overseeing bills and rent responsibilities. She asked them, "'Do you *know* who I am?' I never took a penny. I had a group of people trust me with something. I never took a penny from them. . . . For me, it was that somebody gave me an opportunity. From then, I became president of the house, and then I got to do other things. That was phenomenal for me." She helped organize the Women's Oxford House Conference in Raleigh, North Carolina, and then became part of the very first World Council for Oxford House. She began opening Oxford Houses, thirteen altogether. After a few years her probation officer let her know that she had completed her two thousand hours. "I still didn't stop. What started as a real manipulative move on my part turned into being the one thing that changed my life. Who knew?"

In order to open a new Oxford House, the founder of that house has to live on the premises. Julie would apply for a loan for the first and last months' rent according to guidelines and terms set up by the Oxford House nonprofit corporation and the lender, Ecumenical Ministries. Once the loan was secured, she would look for a house to rent by reaching out to landlords and attending community and neighborhood meetings. She was a few years into her sobriety when her ex-husband called and begged her to take the girls back. They were teenagers by this point, and he had younger children as well. The thought of living as the only adult in an apartment with her two teenage daughters was scary to Julie. She was accustomed to living in community with other adults, but this seemed harder somehow. Oxford Houses are organized around geographical chapters, with five or six houses comprising a chapter. The house presidents met monthly to discuss plans and issues that arose. Julie pitched the idea of opening a women and children's Oxford House, the first in the state, and they backed up her idea. She thought that the transition to living with her daughters would be smoother this way, and that eventually she would be okay on her own.

The first women and children's Oxford House was a success. Although families living together created more opportunities for conflict and friction than single adults, and although many of the mothers and children were just emerging from traumatic situations, she remembered it as being a very nurturing and loving environment. Her girls learned a great deal about getting along with others and the value of chores. They lived in the house for about a year, at which point Julie began thinking about moving back to Minnesota. She was off supervision, her parents were aging, and in her opinion, "they had suffered enough sleepless nights wondering if I was okay." She and the girls moved back in 2000. She pursued the idea of opening another Oxford House, and although she opened another one briefly in St. Paul, she found that the sober house business in the Twin Cities was too big for an Oxford House to compete with. The influence of the Minnesota Model created a system whereby sober houses were an extension of inpatient rehab, with a house manager who was in charge of directing and monitoring residents. Sober houses fell under the guidelines and the purview of group residential housing (GRH) grants, funded in part by the state.[14]

Although Julie's passion was in the Oxford House philosophy and organization, her work life since sobriety had always been in a corporate setting. She worked for a company that conducted inventories in privately traded companies. She was good at her job, but she hated it. Over the years, colleagues would share struggles they were having in their personal lives, and she always offered an ear, advice, and support. This happened so frequently that one day she wondered what she was doing at a job she didn't like when people could be paying her for advice. She went to school to become a licensed alcohol and drug counselor (LADC) and earned a bachelor of science degree in human services from Metropolitan State University.

Being inside the criminal justice system and experiencing the trauma, humiliation, and stigma associated with years of chaotic drug use deeply influenced Julie's career in drug treatment. She was particularly interested in the role trauma played in substance use disorders. "It doesn't matter what substances people are using. It is *why* people use substances in the first place." We spoke again about Gabor Maté at this point, because I wondered how she reconciled her loving, secure childhood with Maté's idea that early trauma and addiction were inextricably linked. "I believe that [addiction] is trauma related, that it's trying to relieve some kind of pain. For me it was really kind of the abandonment, the not being good enough for my husband. Did he really love me? [It's] when you start questioning, am I enough?"

After being both a client and a provider in many abstinence-based treatment programs that had punitive responses to relapse, she grew weary of rules that were not working for people who had experienced trauma at any point in their lives.

If the choice was between "let's see what we can catch people doing" versus "what can I do to help you with what is happening in your life today?" she chose the latter. Urine drug screens frustrated her to no end. Clients snuck in microwaved, hot pee that belonged to other people, and in one case, poured Mountain Dew in the specimen cup. She told that client, "If you had peed those bubbles out, you'd be screaming!" Requiring a bodily fluid from someone doesn't prove wellness. "It creates a barrier, and I want to reduce barriers. If I say, 'Here. Go pee in this cup for me,' I just created some anxiety." And anxiety was not the only issue for clients.

One client she had been working with for years had significant post-traumatic stress related to bodily fluids and bathrooms. She even transferred her records so she could remain a client with Julie at her new employer, a suburban methadone clinic. Although the client had been on methadone for years, federal and state laws require regular drug screens. She thought that federal law required eight per year as compared to the twelve the state of Minnesota required. Every time a urine analysis would come up, the woman would go into crisis mode, so Julie let her skip a few. Skipping a few like this did not go over well with her employer who strictly adhered, understandably, to state guidelines that demanded one urine screen a month. "I think partly why she clung to me was not because I was saying, 'You don't have to UA today,' but because I was saying, 'I'm not going to traumatize you again.' She would come in and say, 'I'm using but I'm not going to UA. I can't do that.'"

Similarly, a young male client had a history of severe abuse and couldn't urinate in front of anyone, which was a requirement—someone had to be present while he filled the cup—and then he would end up in a ball on the floor crying. Some of the staff believed he was doing this to be able to sneak adulterated urine into the bathroom. Julie didn't. Although she understood why the law was there, and that using other substances on top of methadone can be dangerous and deadly, she just couldn't comply when she knew clients' past histories of trauma. "There has to be another way."

After several years as an addiction counselor, she decided to work in mental health because in those organizations she found "more harm reduction and a little more compassion." She worked for South Metro Human Services as part of a community treatment outreach team that went to clients wherever they were. She was the first LADC to join them and became part of what they called integrated dual diagnosis treatment, dealing with both mental illness and addiction. For the first time in her career, she saw a model that fit with her own intuitive, person-centered approach. In 2015, she started dreaming about how she could use a similar approach with clients who were part of "a very damaged population with great need and lengthy, chronic substance abuse." Very specific experiences led her to open a treatment center for the people she witnessed and the person she had once been: someone hanging on for dear life at the bottom of the social ladder, among those most scorned and incarcerated for their struggles with life, mental illness, addiction, and homelessness. The seeds of Resurrection Recovery were sown.

When considering names for her center, she remembered a plant that she'd heard of, the resurrection plant, also called the Rose of Jericho, and decided on Resurrection Recovery to symbolize the rebirth she hoped to foster among her clients. It isn't a particularly attractive plant when it is stressed and dried up, but its ability to blossom into green, to come back to life after existing in waterless, inhospitable conditions, resonated with her. After listening to Julie's story, I saw that she, too, was a Rose of Jericho who had thrived and restored herself after so much personal loss and deprivation.

When we met in her offices in 2017, I understood some aspects of what she intended to do and who she was focused on as clients, but exactly how committed she was to serving people experiencing homelessness only became abundantly clear when I took a look at her website. No other inpatient or outpatient drug treatment website that I had ever seen had a mission that read like hers: "Resurrection Recovery's mission is to provide individualized treatment for men and women who experience chronic homelessness, substance use and co-occurring mental health issues with the goal of improving their health, well-being, and quality of life." Chronic homelessness was listed before substance use disorder? And on the home page, "We employ a holistic, non-threatening, harm reduction approach to meet each individual's complex needs."[15] The connection between homelessness, mental illness, and substance use disorders has long been established—in fact, these conditions work in tandem. Yet people experiencing these continue to be blamed for their lack of initiative and moral strength.

Looking back on her own experience and now from the vantage point of a treatment provider, Julie offered critique along with a different approach. "Look at how many lives are just shattered all because of that . . . the SWAT team and the guns and all that stuff." She envisioned an approach she'd seen in other countries, one that was humane, one that said, "Let's pull you in, let's sit down with a team full of people, a doctor, an addiction specialist, a mental health specialist and find out what we can do to help you." Instead, she said, more often the experience among her clients is "still this War on Drugs that is literally a war on drug addicts."

Paula DeSanto
Minnesota Alternatives/Mental Health Resources, Minneapolis, St. Paul, and Brooklyn Center, Minnesota

It is long gone now, but Paula DeSanto grew up in a home located on the grounds of the Rochester State Hospital in Rochester, Minnesota, where her father, Eduardo Santos, came from the Philippines to complete his medical residency at Mount Sinai in Minneapolis in 1956. While there, he began dating Paula's mother, Sally Sussenguth, who was working as a secretary. They married in 1959. When her father finished his residency, he was hired at the state hospital to be the resident general physician. The campus was "open" then and more of an asylum, so "the patients were free to roam about." Since they lived on the grounds, she and her sisters would go to events in various hospital buildings. Paula came to think of the whole place as part of her home, so much so that she recalled a story her mother tells that one day as a little girl they came upon a terrible mess in one of the hospital bathrooms and Paula exclaimed, "I am not cleaning this up!" Her mother explained she wouldn't have to do that, much to Paula's relief. She has memories of her father, a staff physician (not a psychiatrist), bringing patients home. Some had cuts on their arms. She was curious about why they would do things like that to themselves. She described a culture of compassion in her childhood home that when combined with the experience of living where she did, "set a clear impression that people with mental illness are people that are in trouble and aren't to be feared or aren't pathological or somehow different from us."[16]

The second oldest of five girls, Paula described herself as independent, willful, and good at negotiating. One story she shared stands out. In seventh grade she bought some pot to share with some friends at a movie later. It was in her lunch bag. At some point during the day, the girls were caught smoking cigarettes in the bathroom, and the teacher discovered the pot. Paula was sent to the assistant principal's office where he said he was going to call her mom. "Let me call her," she asked.

> I got on the phone with my mom, and she was a very rational person. She said, "What's going on?" "I'm in the principal's office. I got in some trouble." She said, "Smoking in the can?" I said, "Worse." "Drugs?" "Yep." She came and picked me up, and I was just sent home for the day. There actually weren't any consequences from the school except that they wanted me to be evaluated by a counselor for drug and alcohol problem.

That night instead of going to the movies with her friends, Paula and her dad played tennis. She told her parents it was experimental, that she wanted to be cool so she bought it. They were all going to try it; she didn't have a problem with drugs. Her parents believed her. When the clinic called to schedule an evaluation, she told them she didn't need it and her parents supported her. Neither her parents nor any of her sisters had any interest in or use issues with drugs or alcohol, but following that incident at school, she had a "fairly long-standing experience with cannabis." Due to an enzyme deficit related to her Asian ancestry, she cannot drink alcohol, but she continued to experiment with many other drugs through high school. "I had the good fortune to have enough common sense and supportive home and family environment that I really never got into trouble. I was able to maintain my academics, and I started working at fifteen. . . . I didn't get caught again. Curiously, by the time I graduated high school I pretty much had outgrown most of that stuff."

Early in life, Paula felt pretty sure she would become a lawyer. After earning an associate's degree at Rochester Community College, she transferred to the University of Minnesota to finish a degree in political science. Instead of starting right away, on a whim she decided to use her college tuition money for one semester to go on a road trip to Arizona with a friend. On that trip, "some sort of epiphany occurred to me and I decided I didn't want to be an attorney. Instead I wanted to be a social worker." The desire to be an advocate for people remained, but her focus had changed. While she worked to finish an undergraduate degree in human relationships, she began a job as a mental health worker without having had any prior training in the field. She surmised that she was hired at the two-hundred-bed facility because in the interview she knew the difference between mental illness and mental retardation. She moved up in that position and then went on to get a master's degree in psychiatric rehabilitation counseling from Boston University.

She was drawn to the program because of the work of Dr. William Anthony. In the early 1980s, his ideas about how to care for people with severe mental illness were very progressive. Paula recalled the main concept she learned from Anthony then: "The idea that there's a patient movement out there, that there's an approach toward mental health care that doesn't put the physicians in charge, that it really is the person that should be in the center, and the doctor and the medical team are just one part of that."[17] The patient's goals, wants, and needs should be respected in the care plan and process. This philosophy laid the groundwork for all of her future work helping people manage their mental health challenges, substance use disorder included.

DeSanto developed a new supportive living services program for the organization, and her work became known by people at the Minnesota Department of Human Services. The largest state hospital, Anoka, was building a new facility and wanted to incorporate some of the latest best practices—toward a more person-centered model of care. "My job was to actually close two of the units at the state hospital and open up then two sixteen-bed units, one in Bloomington and one in St. Paul. Then transition the rest of the units to the new facility. Integrate their mental health and substance use disorder care and bring patient-centered state-of-the-art services to the state-of-the-art hospital." She found herself caught in an institutional disconnect, however, between the hospital's desire to integrate patient-centered care and their long entrenched reliance on the public safety medical model for mental institutions. "It was a very difficult system to try to change because everybody's worried about risk and liability."

Five years into this job, she had another epiphany, a dream actually. "I had a dream that if I stayed at that job I was going to get cancer. It was one of those really, really obvious messages and so I listened to the dream." She gave them a full year's notice to wrap up projects, and when she quit, went traveling for six months. Upon her return, she got a job with People Incorporated, "a very mission driven, pretty state-of-the-art mental health organization." She spent nine years there, directing one of their campuses on Minneapolis's North Side. She created an integrated network of services and led a successful capital campaign. She really thought she would end up retiring from that organization. And then she had another epiphany: "It was a Sunday afternoon and I was in the tub and this message said, 'You need to open a drug and alcohol treatment program.' 'What are you talking about?' 'You need to do this.' 'Alright.' There I was. I guess in 2009, April, basically given marching orders. We opened that September and here we are today trying to recreate the system." After hearing about this third epiphany of hers, I asked, "Who would you say your marching orders come from in your epiphany?"

"I think they're just universal."

"Something bigger than yourself?"

"Yes. I think I'm here to provide service and to give guidance. I think that we all have access to that if we tap into that flow and listen—if we're willing to listen and be open."

Asking interviewees about their spiritual or religious background was never on my list of questions, but the topic did come up several times. And in that moment, in her office on a cloudy winter day, something about Paula DeSanto—her clarity of purpose, her generous, open-hearted nature—it begged the question. I was glad I had broached it because then she said, "I appreciate you emphasizing that because I think that probably is what kind of keeps me going. I just trust that we're doing what we're supposed to be doing and we're doing the best we can." And by "we," I knew she meant all of us. She went on, "I just have an enormous confidence that if it all comes tumbling down, then it's time to do something else. My survival doesn't rely on anything. I trust that, regardless, I'll be okay."

So much of the Minnesota Model relied on the peer-to-peer model begun in AA, where people in long-term recovery helped others who were trying to recover. For decades, much of the industry's credibility and authority relied on their lived experiences based on their alcohol and drug addictions. They knew the feeling, the demons, the challenges. Since Paula was not among them, I asked her why it was "that in this field people feel like the person that they're talking to or confiding in has to have had that same experience to effectively relate to and treat them, when in all other aspects of psychotherapy and medicine we don't have that expectation?" She explained that it was embedded in the design of the model, "the system created that phenomenon," and it was unique to drug and alcohol treatment. "If I don't have that personal background, I can't help them? There's no way we can walk in everybody's shoes. What matters more is that we are people who are really interested in trying to help. . . . We're compassionate. We're welcoming. We teach skills."

She had been working to create person-centered mental health services for her entire career and felt discouraged about how little positive change had occurred in substance use disorder treatment, especially when contrasted with how the field of mental health had evolved. "Mental health has made enormous strides toward moving toward a patient-led recovery movement. . . . I think we've come a long way in mental health in terms of making that a rehabilitative experience and much more person-centered. We have a long way to go. But with drug and alcohol we were still stuck in the 1950s."

> I was feeling pretty discouraged about . . . the revolving door . . . a continuous loop, barriers to access, unwelcoming, one size fits all, blaming the family, all the stuff. . . . I saw it firsthand, I heard about it from clients over and over. It's just like, how long are we going to keep blaming the client for the system's failure?

I had heard almost the exact same comment from Dr. Charlie Reznikoff when we were discussing the Minnesota Model. "You can be in Twelve Step programs, but you can only blame the dead person for their death so often before people will just reject it."[18] The system was failing. Paula decided to start her own model that she named the Minnesota Alternatives. Versed for years in program development, networking, and capital campaigns, she decided to start her own program in Anoka County where she had worked for years and was well connected. From the very beginning she was open to letting the model evolve based on feedback from clients. She created the treatment program's structure by drawing from the work of her heroes, some of whom include William Anthony, Gabor Maté, Mark Lewis, Joe Rispenza, David Mee-Lee, and Marsha Linehan. The overriding approach was client-centered in ways she had never seen in traditional drug treatment, and it focused on one central question: What is the client's unique vision for their definition of recovery and what could the team offer to help the client figure out how to get there? This idea is a significant departure from the Minnesota Model, regardless of the extra skills and new therapeutic interventions some facilities have begun to incorporate.

At Minnesota Alternatives, Paula wanted to build in much more substance use disorder–related scientific and educational information for clients about brain development, neuroplasticity, and trauma impacts on addiction. If people needed accountability, which some do, they offered that as well. I asked what she meant by accountability and quickly realized it was not the typical drug and alcohol screens to try to "catch" people. What she meant was accountability more like a coach or a teacher: counselors who work closely with clients to create and track goals and action steps, to make agreements, and if the client desired, drug and alcohol screenings. This form of accountability was based on meaningful goals, mutual respect, and in an environment where it was safe to be honest. This was a very different culture than traditional treatment settings where counselors often function as an extension of probation, and where clients often work to hide their realities for fear of punishment or fear of getting kicked out of a program. "Probation and addiction treatment are in bed together. What's with that? That's just absurd how that developed." I was impressed with the flexibility and trust in what she envisioned. Minnesota Alternatives allowed clients to decide how long they wanted to participate in their programs, and whether they want to be evaluated for medications, including Suboxone and methadone, and worked with those providers to coordinate care. Reducing barriers to care was critical, as was encouraging clients to engage in the parts of the programming that best resonated with them. In most rehabs, inpatient and outpatient, clients have to attend every session/class regardless of how many times they have been in treatment and regardless if it never worked for them. Success equaled working through the first four Steps of the

Twelve Steps in thirty days, attending AA meetings regularly once discharged, and remaining abstinent from drugs and alcohol, including opioid-addiction medications. In contrast, she explained:

> We teach skills on a regular training curriculum, like you would in college. If you demonstrate that if you get this, you're integrating it, then skip [the skills] class that day. You don't need to be there, it's not relevant to you. If you want to go because you want the reinforcement because you learn through repetition, fine. If you want to go because you want to support your peers in learning and be an example, fine. You don't have to. You don't have to do stuff that you already know.

Then she shared something that surprised me: "Ironically, what we find is that people don't want to stop [attending]. We have to push, gently encourage people out." Five years after opening, Minnesota Alternatives opened a nonprofit arm of support services to help clients maintain their new knowledge and plan in a supportive community environment. "As people are getting ready to go and have got it, they've really developed mastery, they have gained or regained control of their lives, then we say, 'Why don't you start dabbling with some support services? Just start going over there while you're still actively in treatment and check out some of the support services.'" Every week night at least one group meeting or activity was available at no cost to participants, all drop-in, with no paperwork needed, and each was led by someone who had received specialized training to do so. They offered coed and gender-specific peer support groups, a family and loved ones group based on CRAFT (Community Reinforcement and Family Training) and a Smart Recovery group; on Fridays, they provided a movie and meal for drop-in social time.[19] Although Minnesota Alternatives does not host an AA group on site, several clients work the Twelve Step program while also attending Minnesota Alternatives, and Paula reiterated, "They're not mutually exclusive."

They were also working with addiction medicine physicians and psychiatrists to be able to prescribe Suboxone for clients who wanted it; they were able to coordinate care with methadone clinics, and often began the whole assessment process with a primary care doctor. Aspects of what she shared began to sound like a harm-reduction approach, and before I could ask, she said, "When people ask, what's your program philosophy, I don't throw out harm reduction because people think all kinds of things when you say that. I say, we are person centered, meaning we embrace a whole range of goals from abstinence to harm and risk reduction." Harm reduction clearly has stereotypes still attached to it, but I was glad she acknowledged its role in their vision of a new system for substance use disorder treatment.

Insurance companies have embraced her new model of care, and I sensed another breakthrough on the horizon related to insurance and how the industry has begun to take notice of alternatives to the dominant model.

> The health insurance companies understand that substance use disorders on the severe end are not episodic, typically, and don't just kind of go away. It's a long distance through the whole process. . . . Generally, people need to have the opportunity to move in and out of services fairly seamlessly if their acuity changes, if their needs change. To have a system [like Minnesota Alternatives] that says, "We'll hang in there with people long term as they go through the ups and downs of their illness and then keep them engaged." The health plans, they're like, "We love that." They're still engaged. It's keeping them from more higher cost services or emergency rooms.

She said that when she began billing in 2009, she did not need to sell her program to insurers—they were thrilled. "Health insurance companies are fed up with everybody getting the same old, same old." She was shocked when she attended a providers' meeting with insurers and no one but Minnesota Alternatives had outcomes data to share with them. They had admissions and discharge data, but no clinical outcomes, no evidence of positive behavioral changes after treatment ended. Before 2016, Minnesota Alternatives showed that 60 percent of clients successfully completed the program, and twelve months later, 90 percent were living again with a reasonable to high quality of life with no problematic drug use.[20]

Paula summarized her vision for a new addiction treatment system by pointing again to the mental health system and the important changes that occurred when counseling and psychotherapy embraced a person-centered approach in the 1950s.[21] It was a long list, but it made a lot of sense now that I was familiar with her background in community-based, person-centered mental health services. She began by pointing out that mental health care has a lot of community-based services and programs, things she would like to see modeled in addiction treatment. I made a list as she spoke:

> Therapists see people long term; you don't cut them off because they have problems with their symptoms. You should be able to see your counselor long term.
>
> You should be able to get wraparound services in your home if you need that level [and] that would include a prescriber and a nurse and a counselor and a therapist.
>
> You have prescribers available to you long term so when your symptoms become more severe they don't cut you off.
>
> If you need outpatient programs, you should be able to move through them fairly quickly without having to go through complex assessments. You should be able to stay engaged with them long term.
>
> A much more robust peer support system with peer support centers.
>
> And have peer outreach workers, too, so that they can go out in people's homes as needed.

She also has a vision of co-located drug and alcohol services that are in general practice clinics, so that someone can just go "right down the hall" with a "warm handoff" from their primary care provider to get information and perhaps an assessment. This seemed similar to what Dr. Bob Levy was doing by offering addiction medicine in primary care clinics, but it expanded the scope and access points. Dropping the assumption that everyone with problematic use will need to go to treatment means that besides saving a huge amount of money, providing a trained mental health and addiction specialist to meet with right away might go a long way toward preventing more severe consequences in the future. "This assumption that if you're in outpatient and you have a use episode that you need residential—that's the most absurd thing I've ever heard." Again, the science versus the entrenched system. Minnesota Alternatives decided to accept goals other than abstinence because "there's this whole theory of cross addiction, that if once you have an alcohol problem, you automatically have an opiate problem. Or if once you have a cocaine problem, you automatically have a cannabis problem. It's not founded. It's inaccurate. It's not based in our neurophysiological capacity."

Our time together was wrapping up. I asked about the book she wrote to share these ideas, and she promptly handed me one to keep. The very first page of *Effective Addiction Treatment: The Minnesota Alternative* acknowledges that Twelve Step–based treatment programs have helped "countless people recover and improve their lives," but that there are some people who have not engaged with this model or found it ineffective. "Alternative approaches are needed." It goes on to describe the need for humanistic and science-based approaches, with humanism being "a democratic and ethical life stance which affirms that human beings have the right and responsibility to give meaning and shape to their own lives." She ends the section by thanking the "many people who work to ensure choice, dignity, and self-determination for those in need."[22]

As I looked briefly at the book, noticing its accessible format, she said something that demonstrated how she truly lives by the statement she'd made only an hour earlier, when she said she thinks she is here—in the big sense, the spiritual sense—to serve and give guidance to others. She said, "I'm not trying to covet this. I want this approach to be available to anybody who wants to try any part of it. I do lots of training. I give information out. I don't require that you go through these high cost trainings in order to use the stuff. I wrote a book that's just very simple. Take it, use any of it, any pieces of it you want. Call me." And then she said that if anyone wants to try it and is afraid, she'd give them some reassurance and tell them "how to cover your butt" if you have concerns. "I'm not guided by fear; I'm not guided by liability or worry." Her philosophy with the entire program is simple and loving: "Let's just do the best we can to create an environment where people feel welcome and comfortable so they can get out of survival mode and start to open up and trust and heal."

The client response to Minnesota Alternatives "has been overwhelming. We cannot keep up. We cannot even come close to keeping up." They were about to increase program capacity at the Spring Lake Park office and were opening another location in St. Paul. Both of those things happened after we spoke. They also hired a full-time psychiatrist for mental health and medication-assisted treatment, who is also working with the Emergency Physicians Professional Association to help them address barriers to initiating Suboxone prescriptions in emergency departments. Livio Health Group, a mobile primary care unit, spends one afternoon per week at the Spring Lake Park location to provide walk-in and open-access care for people seeking help with SUD and in need of primary care.[23] In October 2018, Mental Health Resources acquired Minnesota Alternatives and Paula became vice president of service integration where she worked with staff to better equip them to help clients who have co-occurring mental health and SUD by using a variety of community-oriented strategies.[24] Paula retired from Mental Health Resources in May 2020. When she is ready to move on to another project, one that also helps her fellow human beings, she said she will be working on dignified death/physician aid-in-dying legislation in Minnesota. Looking back at her career and forward to what she aspires to, it is clear that autonomy, trust, and compassion have guided Paula DeSanto's life and work.

Yussuf Shafie
Alliance Wellness Center, Bloomington, Minnesota

Although Somali students and scholars had been settling in the Midwest for decades, the population surged in Minnesota after a civil war broke out in Somalia and the United States began issuing visas to war- and famine-battered refugees in 1992. Most of these refugees settled in Minneapolis and other smaller Minnesota cities via resettlement agencies and nonprofit faith-based Christian organizations. But within about two years, the wider Somali community started to create its own organizations to facilitate migration and services for the new arrivals. The refugees were from rural and urban communities and represented a wide array of vocations—teachers, civil servants, merchants, farmers, entrepreneurs, and students. Minnesota is now home to one of the largest Somali communities in the Somali diaspora, and the Cedar–Riverside neighborhood in Minneapolis has become a hub for hundreds of thriving organizations, mosques, and businesses.[25] The estimated number of East Africans in the state is around 125,000, with 70,000 of those of Somali descent.[26]

The colorful hijabs and jilbabs worn by Muslim women and the traditional tunics and embroidered caps worn by Muslim men are now frequently seen in communities throughout the state, not only in

Minneapolis and its suburbs. Second- and third-generation Somalis have adapted their clothing preferences in innovative and modernizing ways, allowing for sports and athletic activity of all kinds. Despite their successes, Somali immigrants and refugees have not been exempt from discrimination, prejudice, and hate crimes in Minnesota.[27] Somali scholar Cawo Abdi noted that "the community is reaping some of the benefits associated with migration while also becoming entrenched in inner-city, segregated urban America and is thus not enjoying full citizenship."[28] Somali community leaders are working hard to change minds and barriers to success.

Minnesota has a rich civic life that is reflected in one of the highest voter participation rates in the country; this fact no doubt combined seamlessly with the tradition of East African community-mindedness, and before long, local and national politicians emerged from these immigrant and refugee communities. In 2010, Hussein Samatar was elected to the Minneapolis School Board, becoming the first Somali American elected to public office in the United States. Minnesota sent Congresswoman Ilhan Omar, herself a child refugee, to represent Minnesota's Fifth District in 2018, where she was sworn in as the first Somali member of the House of Representatives. The history of East African communities in Minnesota has been documented in several impressive projects, such as oral history collections, museum exhibits, research, books, and community engagement initiatives.[29] I was fortunate to meet one community leader whose mission was to help people struggling with trauma, mental illness, and substance use disorders in the Twin Cities and surrounding suburbs.

Yussuf Shafie's parents moved to Kenya when the Somali civil war broke out in the early 1990s, and Yussuf and his siblings were born there. When he was around eleven years old, his family immigrated and began a new life in Burnsville, Minnesota, a sprawling suburb fifteen miles south of downtown Minneapolis situated on the south bank of the Minnesota River. When they arrived in the United States, Yussuf spoke Swahili and Somali but no English. "I worked really hard, learned English, [and] went through a lot" in middle and high school. His parents valued higher education, and so they expected him to go to college. He had a rough first year at a suburban community college, "playing basketball and chasing girls," but when he learned that his financial aid would be cut if he didn't bring his grades up, he buckled down and stayed in school until he finished a master's in social work.[30]

Laughing, he told me that while he was finishing his undergraduate degree and beginning his master's program, his sister convinced him to go in with her on an African restaurant idea—open and run it together. He agreed, and they opened Tawakal in Burnsville in 2013. The restaurant received great press and the business was going well, but his heart wasn't in it. He told me that despite having neither family nor personal history with addiction, he had been passionate about helping people with mental health and addiction since he was very young. After earning his MSW from the University of Minnesota, he worked for a year at the Community University Health Care Center and learned much more about addiction and mental illness. His supervisor there, Kate Erickson, wasn't surprised to learn that he wanted to start an outpatient treatment center of his own by opening a culturally informed addiction treatment center that focused on East African experiences to directly help his community. She said, "Yussuf is a born overachiever, a unique person with more tenacity than most."[31] I agreed with her, and I was only ten minutes or so into my interview with him. His ability to have a few projects going at once, always looking toward the next good thing to do, was impressive and I wondered where he came by it. Shafie attributed his persistent work ethic to his mother, who had owned a trucking company in Kenya before they came to the United States. It was an uncommon business for a woman to run in the 1990s, and he credited her for creating the drive in him to work hard, take risks, and start new things.

Alliance Wellness Center opened in 2015 in Bloomington, a large, first-ring suburb south of Minneapolis, made famous by the Mall of America. When choosing a name, Shafie told the Minneapolis *Star Tribune* that he didn't want the words "treatment" and "addiction" in the organization's name so as to keep the focus on wellness, and in part due to the entrenched stigma against both drug abuse and mental illness in East African cultures. "Wellness" was also in line with his goal of empowering people in his community to seek help, and he hoped that through his being both Somali and a practicing Muslim that he could build their trust.[32]

When we met at Alliance Wellness Center two years later, community trust was apparently abundant and growing more so. They had a staff of six, a "day group" with a culturally specific focus, and a variety of treatment modalities, such as cognitive behavioral therapy, dialectic behavioral therapy, and EMDR (eye movement desensitization and reprocessing), a simple technique used for healing traumatic memories. Alliance also owns two houses that provide lodging for up to twelve men in the outpatient program. Shafie said supportive housing was of paramount importance for success in his program because so many of his clients were not allowed to go home as a result of their drug or alcohol problems. While clients were in the program, staff tried to helped them find long-term housing options and jobs and, like Minnesota Alternatives, welcomed former clients at group meetings even after they had moved on.

Shafie also incorporates harm-reduction principles in his clinical approach. The topic came up right away when I asked him about treatment approaches and he used a common harm-reduction catch phrase.

I think the most important thing is to meet people where they're at. That's the first important thing. We need to figure out if they have toothpaste. Let's go to Wal-Mart and get them some toothpaste. Let's not worry about the alcoholism or the opioid addiction right now. He needs a towel and some toothpaste and we'll start with that. Let him get some sleep tonight and make sure he brushes his teeth. Dignity is very important.

In a smaller program, he has flexibility that a lot of bigger treatment companies don't, and they also often have policies that keep them from paying close attention to the personal dignity of their clients. He used toothpaste again as an example. "There are big companies out there that have their own policy, 'Our policy is we cannot buy a client toothpaste.' Well, yeah, but that doesn't help anyone if he can't brush his teeth. He's probably afraid to talk to you. . . . I think the most important thing is just treat people like human beings." Pragmatic compassion was what struck me about Yussuf Shafie. Simple and sensible. Toothpaste as an example of a "barrier to care" struck me as a small but powerful symbol of how easy it can be to treat someone in crisis who is alienated from their loved ones with simple gestures to build confidence. This is not to say that all of the other treatment modalities and medical, clinical supports aren't key to recovery, but that such a simple connection to human dignity and worth can make a huge difference in how a person feels when entering an environment where uncomfortable, scary behavioral change is required.

Cultural competence was particularly important with his Muslim and East African clientele, and although he admitted it is a broad term, he couldn't stress enough how important it was for their success in recovery. Many Somali families experienced multiple traumas over a couple of generations related to civil war, famine, and resettlement in a country with starkly different cultural and religious traditions, and more recently, plenty have felt the fear of xenophobic attacks on Muslims as well. When the American-born children and grand-children found themselves living in two very different worlds, as East African Muslims and Americans, the older generations' hold on rigid, long-standing cultural taboos about mental illness and addiction were visibly hurting the younger generation. All cultures have some ta-boos about these problems, but Shafie believed theirs were particu-larly stark and unyielding: "Either you're crazy or you're not. Either you're a drunk or you're not. Either you're a good person or you're a bad person. There's no in between. That's my biggest frustration." The religious requirement of no alcohol consumption made this rigidity even harder to bend. He went on, expressing the baffling nature of this problem. "Because you're a Muslim you're not supposed to drink alcohol; it's forbidden. And I'm like, why do we have fifteen clients in a group right now that are talking about alcoholism and addiction? And they're Muslim. It's like the elephant in the room. The worst thing you could do is drink. It's like being the priest's daughter and get-ting pregnant. It's like the worst thing." Family and community pride made it difficult as well, and he thought this might be a reason why it might be harder for East Africans to enter treatment, especially with him. The community is relatively small—he imagined a young person thinking, "Do I want to get help? Yussuf will know my problem now, and he might know my mom or dad." The pride and shame may be even stronger working with someone from the community, and yet, if they were to go elsewhere, they might not find the same cultural support and understanding.

I knew I wanted to broach it, but I didn't even have to ask how women with addiction fared, because he offered it right up. "People are shunned, and it's pretty bad. Especially for women. You're a woman, you're a person of color, you're a Muslim, and you're an ad-dict. It's the worst thing. You're down on the bottom." Two years after our interview, I got a small sense of what he had been describing, in a YouTube video put together by Somali TV of Minnesota.[33]

A thirty-something Somali Muslim mother in recovery, Biftu Jillo, had been invited to speak at a community event sponsored by Generation Hope, a nonprofit organization formed in 2019 by youth who've lost friends to drug overdoses. They had held their first community meeting in September after four Somali youth died by fentanyl overdose in less than one month. Khadar Abi and Abdirahman Warsame, cofounders of the group, wanted to have open discussions about the problem. "The only reason we are doing this is because we feel like no one would understand or care if we didn't step up to the plate," Warsame said. "Everyone that's part of our organization, including Jillo, has had some kind of experience with substance abuse or gang violence or both. Through our stories and the community's support, everyone can feel our pain too."[34]

Speaking to a mostly East African audience of mothers and youth, Biftu told her own powerful addiction story. Kids played in another part of the gym while the rest of the audience sat rapt, listening to this young woman plead with her community. She sat at a folding table with a few others, including Yussuf. I was relieved and yet not surprised to see him sitting there, offering support. "The Stigma of Substance Abuse for Women" was posted in October 2019, and opens with an older woman holding and comforting Biftu, who is crying.

When Biftu took the microphone, she began a monologue that was direct, brave, and galvanizing. After introducing herself as a recovering addict, a mother, and a Muslim, she jumped right into the damage that stigma and ignorance about drug use was doing to East African families. She took the elders to task, especially. Everyone was listening, and a few people were crying. "I don't know why this community is not taking it serious. We're not blind, we're not deaf. We see how many people we bury every week. And it's mainly due to substance abuse, even the murders. . . . It's serious. . . . And then we think, 'It's not our kid,' until your kid is dead or your kid is in jail." When she asked why the community makes it so hard to get help for drug and alcohol problems, she started tearing up. "Nobody wants to be an addict. Nobody grows up and says, 'Hey, I'm going to be a drug addict when I grow up.' Nobody. We're not losers. We're human beings. We're Muslim, we're alive, we're here." And then she began crying. "But you guys just look at us like we're nobody, like we're not there, like you don't hear us, like you don't see us. Knowing that your sons or daughters are probably just like us, but you don't want to admit to it."[35]

I have attended many kinds of community forums about drugs, and Biftu's testimony was raw, provocative, and pleading in a way that I had rarely seen. Her appeal to parents and elders to listen, pay attention, and love your struggling child took the focus off of individual behavior and addressed a real need for support, not shunning, of young people who struggle with drugs and gang violence. Nothing was off limits. She spoke in particular detail about girls and the painful experiences that often lead them to use substances in the first place. The experiences she recounted were not specific to her community but are unfortunately universal—that is, familiar to young women across the globe, across socioeconomic status, across cultures and religions. It resonated with me.

> Just stop being so tough on the girls. We don't have no magic powers. We are human beings, too. I don't understand why you guys think that we have this power, that we're better. No. . . . The things girls go through? We don't talk about problems in our community. If a girl gets touched by an uncle, or something or whatever, does she go talk to her family? No. She just knows when she's fourteen or fifteen [and tries marijuana] "Oh, I hit this blunt, that feels good, I'm [going to] keep doing that."
>
> Because once you do that you know that negative feeling in your heart stops, so you just keep going, and keep going, and keep going. And then you're just going to see you're lost in it. And when I say lost, I swear to God, it's just that. You feel so lost. You feel so alone, and so miserable. I never wish addiction on nobody. . . . Just make it easy on the girls. Make it easy for them to ask for help.

The audience applauded. Biftu's bravery was fierce.

She admitted that her drug use was something that early on she thought she was in control of. She smoked marijuana and drank alcohol as a teen and then stopped the alcohol but continued with smoking occasionally. She first experienced opioids in the form of pain pills given to her after a dental surgery and discovered that she liked how they made her feel. Years later, after her third child was born, she was diagnosed with Crohn's disease, and a doctor gave her another prescription for oxycodone. "I guess postpartum depression, it just hit me hard. I was getting these pills prescribed anyways. And I just started doubling up on the dose because it makes you feel good. I'm cleaning my house, [I'm] just on point. . . . I found it. This is what it's going to be. And it's from a doctor, so you think it's okay. And it's not. Until you see yourself in that cycle just chasing it."

Biftu also spoke at length about her mother's love and support, and why that was critical for her recovery. "I could come home in any mind-state. My mom would never lock her door. My mom was like a little shelter. She welcomed all the kids. . . . Even boys. She would let them sleep downstairs." All four of her children had substance use problems. Biftu called that heartbreaking and remembered when her mom sat down one day and asked, what did I do? "My mom never touched a drug in her life. She never drank ever in her life, but she still had the heart to understand me and love me and be there for me. . . . I love my mom to death. Without her, only Allah knows where I would be right now." The large audience and the affectionate support captured by the videographer before and after Biftu's talk suggests that the recent uptick in overdose deaths and the stigma about seeking help may have receded a bit since Yussuf and I first spoke in 2017. One of Biftu's last comments highlighted the effort it took to be so open. "I feel better now, but I'm glad I did this. I was really scared to do this. . . . This is needed really bad. And I just wish more people would speak up, and more people would talk."[36] The comments section of the video was full of people praising the strength and courage she had to speak out about the issue.

When I asked Yussuf what his dream was for Alliance Wellness Center five years out, he circled back to one of the first topics we spoke about: housing. The ninety-day limit on housing related to treatment sets his clients up for failure. If clients lose housing and access to resources that help them stay on track before they are secure in their sober lives, a return to drug use is almost certain. One of his goals was to find long-term housing for people who complete his program but don't have a place to live afterward. Shelter for healing from trauma and addiction, at a safe distance and in a space with support, intention, and compassion, is attainable.

Minnesota's history of innovations in medicine, behavioral health, and technology are well known. Creative, compassionate, and dedicated people like Julie Hooker, Paula DeSanto, and Yussuf Shafie are not in short supply in this state, or in this country. Yet I wonder what it will take for us to have the national resolve to provide the kind of consistent care and long-term support that people with substance use disorders need to heal. How many more have to die?

Despite a minor dip in 2017, deaths in Minnesota continued to trend upward and significantly so during the first year of the COVID-19 pandemic. Compared to the first six months of 2019, the same period in 2020 saw opioid overdose deaths increase by 55 percent, and over 80 percent of those involved fentanyl. By the end of 2020, opioid-involved deaths in the state increased 59 percent, with 1,008 people dying statewide.[37] For comparison's sake, in 2016, when I began working on this book, 395 Minnesotans lost their lives to an opioid overdose. And this trend tracks the same nationally. More than forty states raised concerns about the increasing numbers of overdose deaths during the pandemic. During the first three months of 2020, nineteen thousand more people had died of overdoses across the country than in 2019's first three months.[38] If that number continues to rise, it would easily surpass all previous years of data reporting about this epidemic. One positive consequence as a result of the COVID-19 shutdown was the relaxation of previous restrictions regarding take-home methadone doses and video/telephone appointments that changed to allow prescribers the ability to approve patients for buprenorphine medications.

Now more than ever, increasing access to medicine and embracing harm reduction's humanitarian philosophy of "meeting people where they are at" seems not only imperative but certainly among the most positive changes our country could make to lower addiction and death rates. Treating everyone struggling or using drugs with "the dignity, the trust, the love, the belief, and a total nonjudgmental attitude," as harm reductionist Lee Hertel does in his street outreach work, might seem simple, but it would actually be revolutionary.[39]

Conclusion
My Son, Relapsed and Recovered

My daughter Madeleine gets full credit for bringing the man I now consider a son into our lives. At nineteen, she found a loving, gentle, and adaptable partner at an exceptionally tough time in her young adulthood. This book cannot end without including his story. He has personally experienced every single trauma, tragedy, and barrier to success that this book addresses, and remarkably, he has not only survived but has excelled at things he never imagined. He would not brag like this, though. His wise humility and lingering self-doubt sometimes seem indistinguishable, but the delicate scale measuring these traits has kept him grounded for most of the past several years.

The first time I saw Brandon was when we visited our daughter at a treatment center almost a decade ago. She was voraciously reading a Stephen King novel, and he was the friend who had shared his books with her. The next time was later that summer at our house, when he needed a place to store his bike because his sober house wasn't safe. I worried that my daughter was getting into a relationship too soon. And he kind of scared me. He was older, though he looked young, and they shared the same stature. He had a tattoo of a gun on his neck that read "Waiting to Die." That didn't seem promising. He wasn't keen to make eye contact. He was very nervous meeting me, but I didn't know that—I just thought he seemed sketchy and jumpy. It's true. I judged him and I feared him.

For the next few years, they stayed together, toggling between sobriety and active drug use, traveled around the country, and then eventually came back to Minnesota. Shortly after they returned to town with treatment as their goal, another near overdose incident happened, and I put them out of our home in a rage. I felt like ice when I told Madeleine I didn't want to see her again until she had been sober for a few months *or* was calling for a ride to treatment. I screamed at him to leave, using well-placed obscenities. Physically and emotionally, I was raw with anxiety, and yet for many years after that I was ashamed that I had kicked them out, despite the effusive understanding I received from others. My exhaustion, intensified by the surprising commands that blurted from my mouth that night, I would later describe as feeling like my skin had been turned inside out: everything hurt. I had run out of ways to help, lost all trust, and had no more energy left to host the struggles of their death-inviting addiction in our home. They lived in a tent by the Mississippi River for a while. Lucia met up with them, brought them food. I worried myself sick. I stayed awake nights praying for their safety. Seeing them would just break my heart all over again.

One day in early July, Brandon called to tell me he had been approved for a bed in a treatment center the next week, and would I please give him a ride? He also asked if I'd let Madeleine come home. I said I would, yes, but told him not to tell her that. Callous, probably. But I was still desperate for her to go to treatment. *Maybe they won't die in the woods after all.* A few days later, I picked them up at a convenience store and we dropped him off at a clinic for intake. To my surprise Madeleine readily agreed to go to any place where I could find a bed for her. They both stayed in treatment as long as possible that summer, and well into the fall.

Finally, miraculously, tenaciously, they found the right combination of health services, therapeutic programming, and a path to self-care so they could endure the hard journey back to a happy life. They used every tool offered to them and accepted all the supports the state and nonprofits offered, which according to Brandon, was a lot more than most. "I've been on the streets in a lot of the states. I've hit a bottom in every state and tried to reach for help there. Never have I found it except for in Minnesota. Minnesota really picked my ass up and dusted me off."[1] They found a program for stable housing. They worked full time, Brandon finished his GED, my daughter enrolled in college, and together, they expertly and lovingly parented their lively little daughter, born a year after they had initially sought treatment. Creating a stable life like this was new to Brandon.

A lot of the stuff I'm doing today people learn to do when they are eighteen years old. I'm thirty-six. Just now I'm starting to live my life. I've done everything and been everywhere and none of it meant anything because I wasn't really there. I was just a husk of a person until I decided to look around and saw that there is life around me, and I can participate in it in a positive way.

After five years in a stable recovery, Brandon decided he wanted to taper off methadone. He felt secure in his sobriety, he was tired of the lingering side effects and, self-employed as a property manager, the out-of-pocket cost for the medication, even with insurance, was prohibitive, at $147 per week. He took about a year to do it and tapered off completely in August 2019.

A year later, he and I sat together to talk about what happened when he relapsed that fall. What was it about methadone, I wondered? "I felt hindered by methadone. I put pressure on myself to be in the same place in my recovery that Madeleine was. But I had a *much* longer history with drug use and a family history with opioid dependency." He did not realize then how dangerous the decision to taper off might be. Before it got dangerous, though, the side effects from coming off of it, even with the small dose he had been on, were agonizing as they accumulated. The insomnia was horrible. "It felt like I had an electrical charge in my bones, like a vibration." He couldn't sleep as a result and frustratingly knew that all he needed for the buzzing feeling to pass was good sleep, but he couldn't get it. "I did not ask for sleep medication at the time and that was probably a bad idea."[2] Eventually, he got some benzos (benzodiazepine) from someone and tried one. He finally slept. Then the next night he didn't sleep, or the next, so he began to take the pills more frequently. This went on for a month or so.

"At the end of September, one day after work, I made a decision to go get some heroin, and from the moment I made that decision, twenty minutes later, I had a needle in my arm." I had heard stories like this before, and yet it always surprised me. I have finally accepted the fact that I cannot physically or mentally understand what that impulse feels like, especially when a person has so, so much to lose. His child, his partner, his life. What he learned from this relapse was remarkable to hear about a year later, once we had seen him doing well again, thriving again. I asked him if he had any strong feelings about the words that have been declared as stigmatizing by professionals and people in recovery alike, such as "relapse" and "addict." I asked, "Was this a use incident, a slip?" His eyes got wide and he smiled at me. "No. I relapsed!" When he went on to tell the rest of the story, I kept my mouth shut about his use of the word "addict" when describing others. This was his story to tell. I would ask again at the end of our conversation.

He went on. "After I got the dope, I had it in my hand, I was driving and telling myself, 'this is a bad idea, it is not too late, just toss it out the window.' Right then, a wasp flew into my truck and stung me on the fucking eyelid. Nature always does that to me. A beaver, an eagle, and now even a wasp. That didn't even stop me. I kept going. I used it." Brandon is a thoughtful, sensitive man, an avid reader, and a keen observer of people and of the natural world. I did not stop the story to ask about the beaver or the eagle, but I knew what he meant.

From other stories I have listened to, I knew the next thing he said was true for many people while they are actively, intensely using drugs.

> The next thing I knew, honestly, it was a month later, I was sneaking around, moving money from accounts, trying to cover my tracks. I needed to tell somebody what was happening. I was so ashamed. . . . There were so many times I wanted to just blurt it out to my wife, "I've been using!" But I couldn't. I just looked at her and knew how betrayed and hurt she was going to feel.

As he got deeper in, he knew he had to tell someone. One day when he was getting his hair cut by a stylist friend, he told her he was using heroin. He said he was working it out, that he was going to stop. She was too worried and scared about his safety. She called Madeleine, who insisted he get on methadone immediately and said that he had to leave their home. The news was devastating, shocking, scary, enraging. The betrayal, the hiding, the sneaking around—and their daughter. It shattered so much of the trust and work they had done together to build a life.

Brandon called his sponsor, who let him stay at his house, until he realized that Brandon was still using. He asked him to leave but said he would meet him at the clinic whenever he wanted to help him arrange for inpatient treatment. Brandon then spent several days in rural Minnesota, in a place where he knew people who used meth and heroin. Our entire family was thrown back into a place we had not been for a long time. A week later, on a Monday morning, his sponsor met him at the methadone clinic. After Brandon got his dose, he went to the receptionist counter and said, emphatically, "I really need to get into treatment today, today is the day. I am afraid for my life if I don't." The receptionist just looked at him and said he could make an appointment for the next day or the day after because no one was available. They were all in a training, on the premises, but not available. He asked to see the program director, and when that person arrived, Brandon said, "This is the perfect opportunity for someone to be trained in how to help get an addict in serious need of help into a safe place. I might not have tomorrow or the next day." As in, he might be dead. He will never forget the other staff member at the desk, Joe, who said to his boss, "Hey, people don't just come in here and say they need to go to treatment right now lightly." Brandon's counselor was called out of the training, and when he and his sponsor got to his office, the counselor said he couldn't help him today. "But can't you just call one of these treatment centers you have on a list right here, and help me get in?" He replied that he'd have to put it all into the computer system, and his computer was off due to the training. Brandon remembers that he and his sponsor, shocked by this, said at the same time, "Don't we just have to push a button to turn it on?" The guy sighed heavily and turned it on. The first place he called for Brandon had a bed available in two days.

If there is one thing I know now, so much of what happens in our lives depends on the care and intentions of others. In a moment like this, if Brandon had not had the fear of death to insist emphatically for help, if Joe at the desk hadn't pointed out Brandon's desperation, if Brandon's sponsor hadn't showed up for him from the beginning, Brandon might not be with us today. There are so many places in our various addiction treatment systems and bureaucracies where a simple decision, gesture, dismissal, or outright rejection tips the balance between life and death. I knew this place well by now. I had put them out of my house, and yes, everyone I have shared this with sympathizes with me and understands why I did, trying to make me feel better about it, but if my daughter had died that day in May 2014, I would never forget that moment, ever, no matter how lost she might have become in her addiction, no matter how much I had already tried or done.

A small but meaningful moment of redemption occurred for me, but not because I was looking for it. Brandon needed a place to stay for two nights. We agreed to let him stay with us. His sponsor brought him to our house and was the one who picked him up to get his dose the next day. He also agreed to bring him to treatment on the second morning. Brandon slept a lot. He ate dinners with us, though. It was painful to see him in such bad shape so quickly. He had lost weight, his eyes were hollow, and he was jumpy from the meth he had used. He talked with us about how scared he had been, how different it was this time, and that he didn't want to die. It was hard to not cry constantly those two days.

Nearly a year later we could sit and talk about this hard time with clarity and love. A couple of years earlier, the "Waiting to Die" gun tattoo was covered by a stylized wolf; the letters E-V-I-L on his knuckles are now simple black squares. We are at ease with each other talking about hard things, and the honest reckoning has been good for both of us. He is three semesters into an associate's degree to be a licensed alcohol and drug counselor (LADC) at Minneapolis College, where one of the first such programs in the country began decades ago. He is back on methadone and has no plans to get off it. He has a strong support system of friends who are addicts, as he calls them. I asked him again about the word "addict" and about calling his friends that, too. Did it feel derogatory at all?

> I believe if you have to do things every day to make sure you don't use, then I think you are an addict. The people who have a problem with language issues aren't serious drug addicts anyway. If you have had a lot of time using and trying to get clean, you aren't worried about someone calling you an addict. That is "little shit," and it doesn't bother me.

Though I know the history of rhetoric around addiction, and that how we use words has an impact on how we think about things, his blunt honesty is always refreshing.

Much of the purpose of this book has been to focus on destigmatizing and humanely portraying the struggles of people who cope with substance use disorders and the people who love them. Brandon keeps me real, keeps all of this in perspective. He came into our lives in a really tough time, and when I first met him, he was definitely not someone I imagined being so thoroughly integrated into our lives and hearts, but here he was, schooling me kindly with honesty and insight, like so many of the other narrators I had the privilege to meet.

As we were wrapping up, I asked him if he learned anything different this time. I was again surprised by the silver lining of his relapse. He said, "All that knowledge I got when I relapsed, about the drugs themselves and the society around it, the culture of users—I guess I needed it. I was disconnected from it those five years and had no idea how it had changed." What had changed, I wondered? Fentanyl is a big part of it, the wide availability of the drug, and dealers abound. Brandon continued:

> I am an old-school drug addict, and this was the first time I was actually afraid for my life when using. The drugs are so different now than they were even five years ago. They are more potent and go through your system so fast. Six years ago, a dose would hold you for eight hours. Now people need one three or four times a day, and the withdrawal is more of a medical feeling, almost embedded in your bone marrow, gets its claws all the way in there. . . . It is such a moneymaker, too, such a quick turnaround, and it is everywhere—the demand is so high because users need it so much faster.

His last experience in a treatment center, one specifically for opioid users, pushed him to want to be an LADC. I remembered he had told me that when I went to visit him one evening that November. He was noticing things he would do differently if he was a counselor, and he spoke up more when he disagreed with counselors who were not "addicts" saying things that didn't resonate with him or the other guys. "All I see is terrible need. People on heroin now are acting like people that were on meth a long time ago. People are more desperate, okay with being in complete and utter poverty. Suburban heroin addicts used to stay with their parents and use indoors. Now there are suburban white kids living in homeless encampments just to stay high on fentanyl." Brandon's anecdotal observations of the increased availability and potency matched the data in the state health department reports mentioned throughout this book.

Before his relapse, Brandon had been in recovery for five years and had settled into good routines, goals, and practices, but I wondered if he had found any new tools this time. His answer surprised me at first, but it made sense, too. "Being more aware of politics—being more engaged in the world—being more socially aware; these activities take up space and time, and they help me stay part of the world. For so many years, I was trying to shut myself out of the world." He will take a significant pay cut from being a carpenter to helping people recover from addiction, but he knows this is the best kind of job for him.

Several years ago, when he was a guest speaker in my class about the history of drugs and addiction, he told my students, "All these different things that I always wanted to tell myself that I was, I actually am now. I'm actually happy, and I actually care about things. I care about myself and I want to help people. I know that it is an uphill battle but all I can do is the next right thing. That's how I live my life: from one right choice to the next. If I lose sight of that in an instant it will strip me right back to where I was." Indeed, the fall was quick and the price was high. He has had to work hard to rebuild trust in all of his close relationships. Brandon caught himself, though, and knew what he needed to do to get back on track, as quickly as possible, when he had scared himself more than ever before. He had created a support system and also had another family to lean on. The shame was intense, but therapists, social workers, his workplace, and friends help keep him grounded and on his way to feeling whole again. He redeemed himself to himself. That opportunity should be what we offer everyone who struggles with addiction: expertise, empathy, generosity, and the space and time to come back from hell as a whole person, worthy of love, shelter, and promise.

The Minnesota Opioid Project

The Minnesota Opioid Project is a collection of oral history interviews with narrators whose lives have been touched by or whose careers center on opioid use disorders, addiction, recovery, and treatment practices. Starting in 2016, I began with dozens of interviews with parents, siblings, addiction medicine physicians, treatment specialists, social service workers, and harm-reduction advocates across the Twin Cities and other parts of Minnesota, the state internationally regarded as the birthplace of Twelve Step–based alcohol and drug treatment. Selections from a sample of these interviews appear in this book.

The opioid epidemic is ongoing, and therefore a complete historical accounting of it does not yet exist. This oral history collection is undoubtedly missing narratives from individuals and communities who have meaningful, important stories to share. Minnesota residents interested in sharing their story may contact me through the project's companion website. As the collection continues to grow, its ultimate goal is to provide interested readers, policy makers, advocates, and future researchers with access to diverse, complex narratives about our successes and failures as we navigate the opioid crisis in Minnesota. The interviews will eventually be housed in a permanent archive, but until then, more information about the project, this book, and related resources can be found on The Minnesota Opioid Project website: http://mnopioidproject.com.

Acknowledgments

This book would not have been possible without the loving trust of my daughter Madeleine. The fortitude and courage with which she faced her opioid addiction emboldened me to ask hard questions of myself and others, to seek out answers that were neither easy nor obvious, and to reflect deeply on the errors and judgments regarding addiction in our society. My daughter Lucia was a wise, empathic source of encouragement and a steady, guiding light along the way. My husband Andy Wright, a companion of the dearest caliber, believed in me when I doubted myself, encouraged self-care, and kept me laughing. My parents, Richard and Paula Sullivan, and my sisters, Linda Sullivan and Maggie Sullivan, continue to be the most steadfast, loving witnesses to my life, no matter what plans I dream up. For their interest and love, I offer thanks to my brothers- and sisters-in-law, Skip Rhudy, Derek Kusiak, Robin and Dave Wright, and Jeff Wright. The caring generosity of my parents-in-law, Dick Wright and his beloved late wife Diane Wright, will never be forgotten.

For five years, while I grappled with an enormous amount of content and writing decisions, my editor at the University of Minnesota Press, Kristian Tvedten, maintained unflappable enthusiasm for this project's scope and purpose, steered me in the right directions (there were many), and gave generously of his time. He is the first editor I have ever had, and if he isn't the last, his kindness and skill will be what I measure any others against.

The amount of gratitude I have for the first group of mothers and fathers I interviewed is difficult to quantify. The power of their stories and their willingness to be so courageously honest, despite great tragedies and troubles, gave me the motivation to pursue dozens of other narrators who had both professional and personal experiences to share. One mother in particular, my dear friend Katy Oswald, provided a generous grant early on that gave me time to interview narrators and begin writing this book.

Introspection, courage, and tenacity are the words that come to mind when I think of the narrators who make up the Minnesota Opioid Project. I was truly humbled by the power of their stories and their trust in me to do something good with their insights, experiences, and even their greatest sorrows. Their stories are now preserved not only as archival evidence of how Minnesota was affected by opioid addiction but as a testament to everyone who is working tirelessly to end it: Greg Anderson, Thilo Beck, Linda Berry-Brede, Emily Brunner, Bill Cole, Brandon Coleman, Janie Bining Colford, Jamison Danielson, Paula DeSanto, Stephanie Devich, Gloria Englund, Nancy Espuche, Robin Evanson, Adam Fairbanks, Carol Falkowski, Kathie Simon Frank, Rae Eden Frank, Carson Gardner, Lee Hertel, Chuck Hilger, Deb Holman, Janise Holter, Julie Hooker, Chris Johnson, Dean Johnson, Jeff Kazel, Chandra Kelvie, Marisa Krause, Wade Lang, Bob Levy, Lori Lewis, Mary McCarthy, Rose McKinney, Ian McLoone, Kirsten Milun, Richard Moldenhauer, Michael O'Neill, Margarita Ortega, Ann Perry, Kim Powers, Sue Purchase, Charles Reznikoff, Shelley Roberts Gyllen, Star Selleck, Marvin Seppala, Yussuf Shafie, Lorraine Teel, Andrew Tuttle, Verne Wagner, Joe Westermeyer, and Mark Willenbring. The 2017 Harm Reduction History Harvest attendees (if not already listed) include Anne Artino, Mikkel Beckmen, Jules Friedman, Sarah Gordon, Karel Hoffman, Mary Morris, Susan Phillips, Christy Rushfeldt, Brandon Sanford, Gayle Thomas, and Bethany Zeller.

I am grateful for colleagues, readers, and friends who provided feedback on manuscript ideas, drafts, and related digital humanities projects: Nancy Campbell, Dominique Tobbell, Sarah Gollust, Kim Heikkila, Kirsten Delegard, Lauren Martin, Greg Donofrio, Ross VeLure Roholt, Rebecca Wingo, Brooke Schmolke, Aisling Quigley, Liz Jansen, Ginny Moran, Paul Schadewald, Brad Belbas, Herta Pitman, Linda Sturtz, and Katie Phillips. Thanks to two European history of drugs colleagues who agreed to meet a total stranger in 2017: Gemma Blok in Amsterdam and Peter-Paul Bänziger in Zurich. The Oral History Association's 2018 conference, the 2019 Macalester Humanities Colloquium, and the University of Minnesota Program in the History of Medicine Noon Lunch Series provided me with opportunities to share aspects of the manuscript as I developed it, and I thank everyone who participated and asked questions at these events.

Talented students helped me with essential parts of the project: Samantha Aamot and Sara Ludewig (a most amazing oral history team), Aditi Dalela, Zach Mallett, Liam Ummel, and Ashley Vargas. A few others made use of the interviews in their own research projects, helping me see anew how oral histories can improve the world through data, harm-reduction education, and even architecture: Fiona Adams, Rosemary Laine, Clara Motinõ, and Charlie Townsley.

For shared meals, walks, trips, lodging, and friendship, I thank Martha and Greg Archer, Marty Broan and Siri Engberg, Juliet Burba, Theresa Coleman, Margaret Drent, Julia Edelman, Marella Hoffman, Michelle Hoffman, Janise Holter, Catherine Jacquet and Liam Lair, Christie Knapp, Michael O'Neill, Teresa Ordorika, Katy Oswald, Ann Perry and Dean Johnson, Abigail Pribbenow, Sara Tedeschi, John and Nina Tuttle, Suzanne Valdivia, and Dorene Werneke. For welcoming a stranger in their lovely Swiss home in 2017, I thank Andy Tuttle and Susan Tuttle-Laube.

Every book is written in a specific place and time, so I honor and humbly acknowledge that the state where I live is the sacred ancestral land and current home to four Dakota and seven Ojibwe Tribal Nations. Many ideas, dilemmas, and iterations of this book were worked out on the hundreds of walks I took around the Chain of Lakes in Minneapolis, most often Wíta Tópa Bde (Lake of the Isles). I treasure the green spaces in my city and appreciate everyone who tends to them. Other places that provided needed solitude to think and write include the Loft Literary Center Writing Studios, Wellsprings Farm Retreat Center, the Perry–Johnson cabin writing retreats, and the Engberg–Broan time-travel cabin, a treat when I was finally finished.

When Covid-19 shut everything down in March 2020, I wondered how this book would ever be relevant in the midst of a global pandemic. Two months later, after the May 25 murder of George Floyd in Minneapolis, with a raging fury and a broken heart, I questioned again if this book was worth finishing. Anyone I sheepishly admitted this feeling to unanimously responded, "Of course it is. Keep going!" Thanks, and thanks again, to each and every one of you.

Notes

Introduction

1. Pipher, *Reviving Ophelia*; Brown and Gilligan, *Meeting at the Crossroads*; Gilligan, *In a Different Voice*; Orenstein, *Schoolgirls*.

2. Spindler, "The 90's Version of the Decadent Look."

3. Wren, "Clinton Calls Fashion Ads' 'Heroin Chic' Deplorable."

4. One of the most vivid accounts of the pain-pill-to-heroin market is Quinones, *Dreamland*.

5. Menakem, *My Grandmother's Hands*. Menakem added "body" to white privilege, and this simple word made such a huge impact on my thinking about the integral issue of race in this opioid epidemic.

6. One interview frequently leads to another—often called "the snowball effect" among social-science researchers. It is also a method for qualitative research when trying to find and work with underrepresented populations. Atkinson and Flint, "Snowball Sampling."

7. Sullivan, "'What Fear Is Like.'"

8. Although humans have been telling stories since the invention of language, oral-history methods and practice in the United States began in the 1930s when writers and academics recorded and transcribed the life narratives of over ten thousand formerly enslaved African Americans as part of the Works Progress Administration's Federal Writers' Project. Sharpless, "The History of Oral History," 10. See also Oral History Association, "OHA Principles and Best Practices."

9. Hoffman, *Practicing Oral History to Improve Public Policies and Programs*.

10. One book in particular offers rich context and analysis for practitioners conducting intense and trauma-filled oral histories. See Cave and Sloan, *Listening on the Edge*.

11. U.S. Centers for Disease Control and Prevention, "Understanding the Epidemic | Opioid Basics | Opioid Overdose | Injury Center"; Planalp, Hest, and Lahr, "The Opioid Epidemic."

12. Dwyer, "Your Guide to the Massive (and Massively Complex) Opioid Litigation."

13. Wilson et al., "Drug and Opioid-Involved Overdose Deaths"; Minnesota Department of Health, "Preliminary 2019 Drug Overdose Deaths."

14. U.S. Centers for Disease Control and Prevention, "Understanding the Epidemic | Opioid Basics | Opioid Overdose | Injury Center."

15. The national and international press just recently started covering the current opioid epidemic en masse. Between 2015 and 2016 press coverage went from 946 articles on the subject to 17,380. By the end of 2017, more than 29,000 articles had been written on the keyword subject "opioid epidemic." ProQuest Global Newstream Database, searching "opioid epidemic," February 19, 2017, https://www.proquest.com.

16. National Council on Alcohol and Drug Addiction, "That's How"; National Council on Alcohol and Drug Addiction, "All American Girl"; Siegel, "Why Activists Think the Super Bowl's Heroin PSA Is Stigmatizing."

17. Netherland and Hansen, "The War on Drugs that Wasn't"; Siegel, "Why Activists Think the Super Bowl's Heroin PSA Is Stigmatizing."

18. Netherland and Hansen, "White Opioids," 217.

19. Alexander, *The New Jim Crow*.

20. Bridges, "Race, Pregnancy, and the Opioid Epidemic."

21. James and Jordan, "The Opioid Crisis in Black Communities."

22. Netherland and Hansen, "The War on Drugs that Wasn't."

23. James and Jordan, "The Opioid Crisis in Black Communities," 411–12.

24. Minnesota Department of Health. "Opioids: Drug Overdose Dashboard."

25. U.S. Census Bureau, "QuickFacts: Minnesota; United States."

26. Minnesota Department of Employment and Economic Development, "Racial Disparities"; Helmstetter, "Racial Disparities in Minnesota."

27. Alexander, *The New Jim Crow*; Hart, *High Price*.

28. Minnesota Department of Health, "Opioids: Drug Overdose Dashboard"; Minnesota Board of Pharmacy, "Minnesota Prescription Monitoring Program."

29. niin gikenjige Harm Reduction Coalition, "The Eighth Annual Harm Reduction Summit."

30. Gunderson, "'How Can We Prevent the Heart from Breaking?'"; Alexander and Greenfield, "Partnering with Tribal Communities to Promote Well-being & Decrease Opioid Overdose Deaths"; Greenfield, "Opioid Overdose Fatality Reviews."

31. White, "The Birth and Spread of the Minnesota Model," chap. 20 in *Slaying the Dragon*; Spicer, *The Minnesota Model*. Hazelden changed its name to the Hazelden Betty Ford Foundation when the two world-famous treatment centers merged in 2014.

32. White, *Slaying the Dragon*, 261; Foote, *The Crusade for Forgotten Souls*.

33. White, *Slaying the Dragon*, 267.

34. White, *Slaying the Dragon*, 267.

35. Nowinski, *The Twelve Step Facilitation Outpatient Program*; Nowinski and Baker, *The Twelve Step Facilitation Handbook*; Nowinski, Baker, and Carroll, *The Twelve Step Facilitation Therapy Manual*.

36. Alcoholics Anonymous, "Estimates of A.A. Groups and Members as of December 31, 2020."

37. Karlen, "Greetings from Minnesober."

38. Campbell, Olsen, and Walden, *The Narcotic Farm*; Campbell, *Discovering Addiction*.

39. Courtwright, "The Prepared Mind."

40. Frydl, *The Drug Wars in America, 1940–1973*.

41. Erickson et al., *Harm Reduction*, 3–11.

42. Author correspondence with El Alcala, November 15, 2020. Also see Diaz, "Student Saves Life with Naloxone Drug from Macalester History Class."

1. Mothering Addiction

1. Jarmolowicz et al., "Executive Dysfunction in Addiction"; Nixon, "Executive Functioning among Young People in Relation to Alcohol Use."

2. Smith, "Three Heroin Deaths, One Dealer."

3. Nelson, *Parenting Out of Control*; Doepke and Zilibotti, *Love, Money & Parenting*.

4. Bebinger, "Fentanyl-Linked Deaths."

5. Rotskoff, *Love on the Rocks*. Also see Bepko, *Feminism and Addiction*; Irvine, "Codependency and Recovery."

6. Knudsen et al., "Service Delivery and Use of Evidence-Based Treatment Practices in Adolescent Substance Abuse Treatment Settings."

7. Vandenberg-Daves, *Modern Motherhood*; Campbell, *Using Women*.

8. Singh, "Doing Their Jobs"; McKeever and Miller, "Mothering Children Who Have Disabilities."

9. Frye, *The Politics of Reality*, 2.

10. American Society of Addiction Medicine, "ASAM Definition of Addiction"; emphasis mine. The entire definition reads: "Addiction is a treatable, chronic medical disease involving complex interactions among brain circuits, genetics, the environment, and an individual's life experiences. People with addiction use substances or engage in behaviors that become compulsive and often continue despite harmful consequences. Prevention efforts and treatment approaches for addiction are generally as successful as those for other chronic diseases."

11. Travis, *Language of the Heart*; White, "Lessons of Language," 39.

12. Rotskoff, "Sober Husbands and Supportive Wives."

13. Beattie, *Codependent No More*.

14. Nakken, *Enabling Change*.

15. Krestan and Bepko, "Codependency," 64.

16. Schach, "Impact of Nar-Anon Family Support Group upon Family Members of Heroin Addicts"; Bumbalo and Young, "The Self-Help Phenomenon."

17. Schach, "Impact of Nar-Anon Family Support Group upon Family Members of Heroin Addicts," v.

18. Kathie Simon Frank, interview, March 15, 2017. Minneapolis, Minnesota.

19. The daily reading she refers to is from the book by Nar-Anon Family Group, *Sharing Experience, Strength, and Hope*.

20. Ann Perry's entire story about her son Spencer is found in chapter 2, "Prognosis Cloudy."

21. Michael O'Neill, interview, January 19, 2017, Minneapolis, Minnesota.

22. White, *Slaying the Dragon*, 265–70.

23. Linda Berry-Brede, interview, June 24, 2016, Dassel, Minnesota.

24. Musto, *The American Disease*, 54–68; Gowan and Whetstone, "Making the Criminal Addict"; Frydl, *The Drug Wars in America, 1940–1973*.

25. Minnesota Department of Corrections, "Fact Sheet: Substance Use Disorder Treatment Services in Prison."

26. The Addict's Mom is a private Facebook group with more than 35,000 members. They also have a public page, https://www.facebook.com/addictsmom.

27. Kim Powers, interview, July 5, 2016, Minneapolis, Minnesota.

28. "From Statistics to Solutions," https://www.fstsconference.com/; see also OYA Community, https://ouryoungaddicts.com/.

29. Rose McKinney, interview, June 16, 2016, St. Paul, Minnesota.

30. Henderson, *Understanding Addiction*; Travis, *Language of the Heart*.

31. OYA Community.

32. Travis, *Language of the Heart*; Clark, *The Recovery Revolution*.

33. Alcoholics Anonymous World Services, "Twelve Steps—Step One," in *Alcoholics Anonymous Big Book*, 24.

34. Alcoholics Anonymous World Services, "Twelve Steps—Step One," 23.

35. Alcoholics Anonymous World Services, "Twelve Steps—Step One," 24.

36. Janie Bining Colford, interview, June 26, 2016, Chanhassen, Minnesota.

37. Substance Abuse and Mental Health Services Administration, "Naloxone"; Campbell, OD.

38. *An act relating to health; providing for drug overdose prevention and medical assistance; limiting liability; amending Minnesota Statutes 2012, sections 144E.101, subdivision 6; 151.37, by adding a subdivision; proposing coding for new law in Minnesota Statutes, chapter 604A*, in Laws of Minnesota, S.F. No. 1900, Chapter 232, 1–4, passed by the State of Minnesota Legislature, May 7, 2014.

39. Rosenblum, "'Good Samaritan' Law Essential for Drug Antidote to Succeed"; Williams, "Legislative Path to Preventing Heroin Deaths Paved with Tears."

40. Swerdlow, *Women Strike for Peace*; Lerner, "The MADD Mothers Take Charge," chap. 3 in *One for the Road*.

41. Grim, "Minnesota State Senator Chris Eaton to Push Legislation to Reform Heroin Treatment"; Murphy, "Lawmakers Chris Eaton, Dave Baker Talk Opioids after Personal Losses"; Collins, "Son's Overdose Death Drives this Minnesota Legislator's Work."

42. Corkery and Thomas, "Drug Industry Wages Opioid Fight Using an Anti-Addiction Ally"; "Big Pharma Buys Clout in Advocacy Over Opioids."

43. Star Selleck, interview, June 21, 2016, Minneapolis, Minnesota.

44. Lori Lewis, interview, June 18, 2016, Oakdale, Minnesota.

45. Minnesota Department of Human Services, "Minnesota State Targeted Response to the Opioid Crisis."

46. Substance Abuse and Mental Health Services Administration, "Buprenorphine."

47. U.S. Food and Drug Administration, "Vivitrol Drug Facts and Label."

48. Neutkens, "Journey with Pain Pills Often Dead End with Heroin."

49. Boss, *Ambiguous Loss*, 134.

50. Boss, *Ambiguous Loss*, 138.

51. Janise Holter, interview, June 14, 2016, St. Paul, Minnesota.

2. Prognosis Cloudy

1. Ann Perry, interview, July 6, 2016, Minnetonka, Minnesota.

2. A 1997 article critiqued the effectiveness of the D.A.R.E. program: Kersten, "Dare to Ask Whether D.A.R.E. Is Doing Kids More Harm than Good," 17A. See also Wysong, Aniskiewicz, and Wright. "Truth and DARE."

3. Harvey, "Dance at Apple Valley Will Cap Drug Awareness Campaign"; Kersten, "Dare to Ask Whether D.A.R.E. Is Doing Kids More Harm than Good," 17A; Wysong, Aniskiewicz, and Wright. "Truth and DARE"; Substance Abuse and Mental Health Services Administration, "Not Your Mother's Scare Tactics."

4. Dean Johnson, interview, January 20, 2017, Minnetonka, Minnesota.

5. Shelley Roberts Gyllen, interview, August 17, 2017. Ely, Minnesota.

6. Bridge et al., "Clinical Response and Risk for Reported Suicidal Ideation and Suicide Attempts in Pediatric Antidepressant Treatment."

7. White, *Slaying the Dragon*, 449.

8. Spencer Johnson, diary.

9. U.S. Food and Drug Administration, "Timeline of Selected FDA Activities and Significant Events Addressing Opioid Misuse and Abuse."

10. For a detailed chronology of how prescription pain pills led to increased heroin use in the United States, see Quinones, *Dreamland*.

11. Mars et al., "'Every "Never" I Ever Said Came True.'"

12. Rule 25 refers to Minnesota Department of Human Services, "Alcohol, Drug and Other Addictions."

13. Substance Abuse and Mental Health Services Administration, "Medications for Opioid Use Disorder – Executive Summary."

14. Mark Willenbring, email correspondence with author, July 2, 2019.

15. Clark, *The Recovery Revolution*; Narcotics Anonymous, "Regarding Methadone and Other Drug Replacement Programs."

16. Spencer Johnson, Allina Medical records, 62, 76.

17. Nar-Anon Family Groups, http://www.nar-anon.org/.

18. Nar-Anon Family Groups, http://www.nar-anon.org/.

19. Knowlton and Chaitin, *Detachment and Enabling*.

20. Ann Perry, diary, 3.

21. Ann Perry, diary, 3.

22. Karen Casey is the author of fifteen bestselling self-help books, published through Hazelden Publishing. Her first book, *Each Day a New Beginning*, was published in 1981. Translated into ten languages, more than three million copies have been sold.

23. Ann Perry, diary, 3.

24. Ann Perry, diary, 2.

25. Substance Abuse and Mental Health Services Administration, "National Survey of Substance Abuse Treatment Services."

26. Ann Perry, diary, 1.

27. Anoka County Medical Examiner's Report, 2016-MN-011706, April 6, 2016.

28. Dean Johnson, private papers; Spencer Johnson's funeral program.

29. Smith, "Three Heroin Deaths, One Dealer"; Smith, "Twin Cities Heroin Dealer Gets 14 Years for Overdose Deaths of Two Men."

30. Smith, "Three Heroin Deaths, One Dealer."

31. State of Minnesota v. Beverly Nicole Burrell, Hennepin County, MN, Court File No. 27-CR-16-13553, May 20, 2016; State of Minnesota v. Beverly Nicole Burrell, Hennepin County, MN, Court File No. 27-CR-16-18602, July 13, 2016; State of Minnesota v. Beverly Nicole Burrell, Hennepin County, MN, Court File No. 27-CR-16-27585, October 21, 2016.

32. LaSalle, "An Overdose Death Is Not Murder," 28.

33. Smith, "Three Heroin Deaths, One Dealer," and Collins, "It's an Opioid Overdose Death. But Is It a Murder?"

34. Collins, "It's an Opioid Overdose Death. But Is It a Murder?"

35. Mullen, "Read Victim Impact Letters about Twin Cities Heroin Dealer Beverly Burrell."

36. MPR News, "Beverly Burrell Delivers a Statement and Is Sentenced."

37. MPR News, "Beverly Burrell Delivers a Statement and Is Sentenced."

38. MPR News, "Beverly Burrell Delivers a Statement and Is Sentenced."

39. Peltier was a Marine veteran who struggled with post–traumatic stress disorder from his two tours in Iraq. His struggle with opioid addiction was described by his mother as a way he coped with PTSD. Choi, "Maplewood Woman Sentenced to 8 More Years in Opioid Overdose Death."

40. Ann Perry, "Trial Discussion," August 16, 2017, Ely, Minnesota.

41. Ann Perry, text messages pulled from Spencer Johnson's cell phone, August 2017.

42. Robert Levy, interview, January 13, 2017, Robbinsdale, Minnesota.

43. Julie Hooker, interview, February 2, 2017, St. Paul, Minnesota. For more on the brain-drug response, see Sheff, Clean, 11.

44. Midwest Medical Examiner's Office, June 2, 2016, "Press Release of Prince Rogers Nelson's Cause of Death."

45. Seth et al., "Overdose Deaths Involving Opioids, Cocaine, and Psycho-stimulants—United States, 2015–2016."

46. Patty Wetterling, as quoted on Spencer Johnson's funeral program, 2016. Wetterling made this statement on November 3, 2015, when new information led investigators to announce they had found a person of interest in the unsolved abduction of her son Jacob Wetterling in 1989. Marnati, "Wetterling Family Speaks Out on Arrest of 'Person of Interest.'"

47. Ann Perry, impact statement, June 21, 2019.

48. Ann Perry, impact statement, June 21, 2019.

49. Dean Johnson, impact statement, June 21, 2019.

50. Dean Johnson, impact statement, June 21, 2019.

51. Shelley Roberts Gyllen, impact statement, June 21, 2019.

52. Shelley Roberts Gyllen, impact statement, June 21, 2019.

53. WCCO CBS Minnesota, "Beverly Burrell to Receive No Additional Prison Time for 2 More Heroin Deaths."

3. Prescription for Humility

1. Booth, *Opium.*
2. Kuhn et al., *Buzzed,* 239.
3. Courtwright, *Forces of Habit.*
4. U.S. Centers for Disease Control and Prevention, "Understanding the Epidemic | Opioid Basics | Opioid Overdose | Injury Center."
5. Wailoo, "OxyContin Unleashed," chap. 5 in *Pain*; Courtwright, *The Age of Addiction,* 232–35.
6. Campbell, Olsen, and Walden, *The Narcotic Farm,* 12.
7. Campbell, Olsen, and Walden, *The Narcotic Farm,* 18.
8. National Institute on Drug Abuse, "Opioid Overdose Crisis."
9. Courtwright, "The Prepared Mind," 258.
10. Frydl, *The Drug Wars in America,* 1940–1973, 332.
11. Frydl, *The Drug Wars in America,* 1940–1973, 326–32; Courtwright, "The Prepared Mind."
12. Clark, *The Recovery Revolution*; White, *Slaying the Dragon.*
13. O'Connor, Sokol, and D'Onofrio, "Addiction Medicine," 1717–18; Wood, Samet, and Volkow. "Physician Education in Addiction Medicine," 1673–74.
14. Mark Willenbring, "Oral History Interview 1," May 17, 2017, St. Paul, Minnesota.
15. Clark, *The Recovery Revolution,* 185–86.
16. Narcotics Anonymous, "Regarding Methadone and Other Drug Replacement Programs"; White, "Narcotics Anonymous and the Pharmacotherapeutic Treatment of Opioid Addiction in the United States."
17. White, "Narcotics Anonymous and the Pharmacotherapeutic Treatment of Opioid Addiction in the United States." 4.
18. White, "Narcotics Anonymous and the Pharmacotherapeutic Treatment of Opioid Addiction in the United States," 32.
19. Fred Ohlerking, director of Care Plus Services, Hennepin Healthcare – HCMC, email correspondence with author, 2019.
20. Charles Reznikoff, interview, January 17, 2017, Minneapolis, Minnesota.
21. Earnshaw, Smith, and Copenhaver. "Drug Addiction Stigma in the Context of Methadone Maintenance Therapy," 112.
22. James and Jordan, "The Opioid Crisis in Black Communities"; Childress, "How the Heroin Epidemic Differs in Communities of Color."
23. Charles Reznikoff, email correspondence with author, August 15, 2017.
24. Robert Levy, interview, January 13, 2017, Robbinsdale, Minnesota.
25. O'Connor, Sokol, and D'Onofrio, "Addiction Medicine"; Wood, Samet, and Volkow. "Physician Education in Addiction Medicine."
26. Parekh and Childs, *Stigma and Prejudice,* 152.
27. Bänziger and Blok, "'Junkie Kingdoms.'"
28. Thilo Beck, interview, February 16, 2017, Zurich, Switzerland.

29. Savary, Hallam, and Bewley-Taylor, "The Swiss Four Pillars Policy."

30. Andrew Tuttle, interview, February 16, 2017, Wettingen, Switzerland.

31. Emily Brunner, interview, June 28, 2017, St. Paul, Minnesota.

32. Dr. Pat Gibbons passed away in 2014 after a brief illness. Schwartz, "A Terrible Loss for Dawn Farm and the Field"; Gavin, "UMHS, Addiction Community Mourn Death of Patrick Gibbons."

33. Hazelden Betty Ford Foundation, "Frequently Asked Question about Medication-Assisted Treatment for Opioid Addiction," http://www.hazeldenbettyford.org/treatment/models/mat-faq.

34. Spicer, *The Minnesota Model*, 130.

35. Marvin Seppala, "Oral History Interview 1," November 6, 2018, Minneapolis, Minnesota.

36. White, *Slaying the Dragon*, 380.

37. "Dr. Donald is this eccentric, old physiologist. He was trained as a veterinarian, but he became a physiologist and helped invent the heart-lung machine. John Shepherd was the president of the American Heart Association at the time and he was on the board of governors and the board of trustees at the Mayo Clinic. He was really one of the top administrators, the top docs in the whole place, and famous worldwide for research."

38. Marvin Seppala, "Oral History Interview 2," January 23, 2019, Minneapolis, Minnesota.

39. Obermeyer, "Prozac and the Great U-Turn in American Psychiatry"; Shorter, *A History of Psychiatry*; Slater, *The Drugs that Changed Our Minds*.

40. By "only medicine available," Marv meant the only medication for opioid use disorder that could be given by a prescription outside of methadone, which is so highly regulated that only certain sites are allowed to prescribe it and clients have to come to the premises to get their daily dose.

41. "Comprehensive Opioid Response with Twelve Steps," brochure, Hazelden Foundation, 2013.

42. Klein and Seppala, "Medication-Assisted Treatment for Opioid Use Disorder within a 12-Step Based Treatment Center."

4. Women of Substance

1. Beck, "100 Years of 'Just Say No' Versus 'Just Say Know,'" 31–32. Claire Clark's chapter, "Selling a Drug Free America," in *The Recovery Revolution* is essential reading for this era in the history of drug-prevention efforts in the United States.

2. Campbell, OD, chap. 12, "Overdose and the Cultural Politics of Redemption," 282–305.

3. Campbell, OD, chap. 7, "'Any Positive Change': Naloxone as a Tool for Harm Reduction in the United States," 149–70.

4. Des Jarlais et al., "Regulating Controversial Programs for Unpopular People."

5. Springer, "Effective AIDS Prevention with Active Drug Users"; O'Hare, "Merseyside, the First Harm Reduction Conferences, and the Early History of Harm Reduction"; Newcombe and Parry, "The Mersey Harm-Reduction

Model"; National Harm Reduction Coalition, "Harm Reduction Principles," https://harmreduction.org/about-us/principles-of-harm-reduction/.

6. Springer, "Worker Stances for Clients Who Use Drugs."

7. Lee Hertel, Harm Reduction History Harvest Transcript, 2.

8. Rae Eden Frank, interview, January 31, 2017, Maplewood, Minnesota.

9. Campbell, OD; Erickson et al., *Harm Reduction*; O'Hare, *The Reduction of Drug-Related Harm.*

10. Sue Purchase, "Oral History Interview 1," April 27, 2017, Minneapolis, Minnesota.

11. Levine, *School Lunch Politics.*

12. Booth Memorial Hospital Oral History Records, University of Minnesota Libraries, Social Welfare History Archives. For an early history of the Booth Brown House, see Heikkila, "'Everybody Thinks It's Right to Give the Child Away.'"

13. Deb Holman, interview, May 19, 2017, Duluth, Minnesota.

14. Clark, *The Recovery Revolution*, 10–11.

15. Amodeo, "The Addictive Personality."

16. WCCO-TV, "Hennepin Avenue, 1978."

17. Morain, "Needle Exchange Programs Can Prevent AIDS."

18. Shullenberger, "Needle Exchange Programs Will Not Prevent AIDS," 138.

19. Extensive documents about AIDS activism in Minnesota can be found in the Tretter Collection, University of Minnesota, Minnesota AIDS Project boxes.

20. Crosby, "Obituary: Toni St. Pierre Blazed Trail for Girls' Sports."

21. Dan Bigg, founder of the Chicago Recovery Alliance, died on August 21, 2018. Keilman, "Dan Bigg Remembered as 'Revolutionary' for Approach to Heroin Crisis, Pioneered Life-Saving Naloxone, Needle Handouts."

22. North American Syringe Exchange Network: https://www.nasen.org/. A safe injection kit includes syringes, alcohol wipes, sharps containers, cookers, and cotton.

23. WAP and Access Works files, collection of the author.

24. Springer, "Worker Stances for Clients Who Use Drugs."

25. Springer, "Effective AIDS Prevention with Active Drug Users."

26. Northern Sun, "About Northern Sun," https://www.northernsun.com/aboutus.html: "Northern Sun got its start back in 1979, right before radiation started leaking from the Three Mile Island nuclear plant in Harrisburg, Pennsylvania (March 28, 1979). Riding a bicycle and carrying a backpack full of t-shirts, etc., Scott (the owner) began selling message-oriented items at anti-nuke events. In 1980, Ronald Reagan was selected President, creating a big demand for anti-war stuff. G W Bush was good for business, too."

27. Sue Purchase, "Oral History Interview 2," May 9, 2017, Minneapolis, Minnesota.

28. Edwards, "Needle Exchange"; Hevesi, "Dave Purchase Dies at 73; Led Early Needle Exchange."

29. ASP Plastics, "Our History," http://www.aspplastics.com.au/our-history/: "1989—partnered with New South Wales Health in the design of the

world's first personal sharps container. This initiative was to become the first of over 150 in the fight against the spread of blood borne viruses."

30. Novotny et al., "The Minnesota Pharmacy Syringe Access Initiative," 22. 2020 Minnesota Statutes, "151.40 Possession and Sale of Hypodermic Syringes and Needles," https://www.revisor.mn.gov/statutes/cite/151.40. MN Dept of Health, "Minnesota Pharmacy Syringe/Needle Access Initiative," https://www.health.state.mn.us/people/syringe/mnpharmacy.html.

31. StreetWorks continues to serve unhoused youth in Minneapolis and remains the strong, collaborative effort of a dozen diverse agencies that provide housing and services for youth: https://www.streetworksmn.org/.

32. "Pride Still Stands Out as Site Tailored to LGBT Clients," 1–1.

33. Edwards, "Needle Exchange"; "Needle Exchange for Addicts Wins Foothold Against AIDS in Tacoma"; Des Jarlais, "Harm Reduction in the USA."

34. Hevesi, "Dave Purchase Dies at 73; Led Early Needle Exchange."

35. Rae Eden Frank, email correspondence with author, August 4, 2020.

36. "Sixth Annual Harm Reduction Summit: Addressing HCV, HIV, TB, STI and Drug Use in Tribal and Rural Communities," conference program brochure, May 2017.

37. Greg Anderson, interview, May 18, 2017, Duluth, Minnesota.

38. "Alcohol Allowed Here," 1–1.

39. Deb Holman, personal Facebook page, July 19, 2020.

40. Sue Purchase, "Oral History Interview 3," May 30, 2020, Duluth, Minnesota.

41. Minnesota Department of Public Health, "HIV Outbreak Response and Case Counts."

5. Dissecting Stigma

1. I was disheartened to find this 2016 study, Creedon and Lê Cook, "Access to Mental Health Care Increased but Not for Substance Use, While Disparities Remain," about the impact of expanded access to substance use and mental health treatment through the Affordable Care Act, that revealed that although mental health services increased, substance use treatment numbers stayed relatively consistent with pre-ACA admissions. And while the ACA envisioned decreasing barriers to care for underinsured people of color, that did not happen either: the authors found that coverage expansion had not helped groups who had historically lagged far behind in access to behavioral health care.

2. Gowan and Whetstone, "Making the Criminal Addict," 69.

3. Levine, *Refuge Recovery*; Glasner-Edwards, *The Addiction Recovery Skills Workbook*.

4. Richard Moldenhauer, interview, March 30, 2017, St. Paul, Minnesota.

5. Solon and Maté, "The Biology of Loss."

6. "Similar to phantom limb pain, when the memory is triggered the motor and somatosensory cortices fire in patterns that are the same as if the actions were actually occurring currently." Midwest Center for Trauma and

Emotional Healing, "Adaptive Internal Relational (AIR) Network Model: An Overview."

7. Maté, *In the Realm of Hungry Ghosts*, 1–3.

8. Maté, *In the Realm of Hungry Ghosts*, 38.

9. Julie Hooker, interview, February 2, 2017, St. Paul, Minnesota.

10. Clark, *The Recovery Revolution*, 10–11. Clark's book traces the history of Synanon from its small recovery community beginnings to its more formal implementation as a behavioral treatment approach in drug-treatment institutions across the country.

11. Julie's opinion of methadone at that time reiterated other common perceptions of methadone as not being a "true recovery" from drugs, as keeping one "hooked," especially among poor and marginalized groups; it was considered just another way to be monitored and controlled by the state. More on this topic can be found in Trysh Travis's article, "The Intersectional Origins of Women's 'Substance Abuse' Treatment."

12. White, *Slaying the Dragon*, 489–90.

13. A great segment about Oxford House aired on 60 *Minutes* on May 5, 1991, and is available at the Oxford House website: https://oxfordhouse.org /userfiles/file/oxford_house_video.php. More about the Oxford House model: Jason, Ferrari, and Davis, *Creating Communities for Addiction Recovery*.

14. Minnesota Department of Human Services, "GRH Basis—Drug/ Alcohol Addiction."

15. The Resurrection Recovery website is no longer available but can be viewed through the Internet Archive, https://web.archive.org/web/2019* /resurrectionrecovery.com.

16. Paula DeSanto, interview, January 26, 2017. Spring Lake Park, Minnesota.

17. Anthony et al., "Efficacy of Psychiatric Rehabilitation"; Anthony, Cohen, and Farkas, "The Future of Psychiatric Rehabilitation"; Anthony, "A Vision for Psychiatric Rehabilitation Research."

18. Charles Reznikoff, interview, January 17, 2017, Minneapolis, Minnesota.

19. Meyers et al., "Community Reinforcement and Family Training (CRAFT)"; Horvath, "Smart Recovery®"; Kelly et al., "From Both Sides."

20. Paula DeSanto, email correspondence with author, July 2020.

21. Rogers, *Client-Centered Therapy*; Raskin, *Contributions to Client-Centered Therapy and the Person-Centered Approach*.

22. DeSanto, *Effective Addiction Treatment*, iv.

23. Livio, https://www.liviohealth.com/ (accessed July 16, 2020): "Livio is a mobile healthcare provider, addressing common, urgent and complex care issues by creating pop-up clinics in nontraditional care settings, partnering with community partners, and delivering in-home care to patients in need." "We work with specific health insurance companies and facilities to provide our services to their members."

24. Paula DeSanto, email correspondence with the author, June 25, 2019. Mental Health Resources, http://www.mhresources.org/mission-history.

25. Wilhide, "Somali and Somali American Experiences in Minnesota."

26. Minnesota Compass, "Somali Population"; Wilhide, "Somali and Somali American Experiences in Minnesota."

27. Paris, "Militia Members Plead Guilty to 2017 Minnesota Mosque Bombing"; Yussuf, "Goodbye, St. Cloud. I Love You, But I Can't Stand the Hate."

28. Abdi, "The Newest African-Americans?," 20.

29. Ibrahim, *From Somalia to Snow*; Roble and Rutledge. *The Somali Diaspora*; Warfa et al., "Somalis + Minnesota"; Wilhide, "Somali and Somali American Experiences in Minnesota"; Yusuf, *Somalis in Minnesota*.

30. Yussuf Shafie, interview, December 19, 2017, Bloomington, Minnesota.

31. Koumpilova, "Somali Social Worker Opens Substance Abuse Treatment Center Aimed at African Refugees."

32. Koumpilova, "Somali Social Worker Opens Substance Abuse Treatment Center Aimed at African Refugees."

33. Somali TV Minnesota, "The Stigma of Substance Abuse for Women, by Biftu."

34. Ibrahim, "'Monster in Our Community.'"

35. Somali TV Minnesota, "The Stigma of Substance Abuse for Women, by Biftu."

36. Somali TV Minnesota, "The Stigma of Substance Abuse for Women, by Biftu."

37. Giesel, DeLaquil, and Wright, "Drug Overdose Deaths among Minnesota Residents from January through June 2020"; and DeLaquil, Giesel, and Wright, "Preliminary 2020 Drug Overdose Deaths."

38. Baumgartner and Radley. "The Spike in Drug Overdose Deaths during the COVID-19 Pandemic and Policy Options to Move Forward"; Zarefsky, "As COVID-19 Surges, AMA Sounds Alarm on Nation's Overdose Epidemic."

39. Lee Hertel, Harm Reduction History Harvest Transcript, 2.

Conclusion

1. Brandon Coleman, "Oral History Interview 1," October 26, 2016, St. Paul, Minnesota.

2. Brandon Coleman, "Oral History Interview 2," August 1, 2020, Minneapolis, Minnesota.

Sources and Bibliography

Oral History Interviews
All oral histories conducted by Dr. Amy Sullivan unless otherwise noted.

Anderson, Greg. May 18, 2017. Duluth, Minnesota. 11 pages.

Beck, Thilo. February 16, 2017. Zurich, Switzerland. 19 pages.

Berry-Brede, Linda. June 24, 2016. Dassel, Minnesota. 31 pages.

Brunner, Emily. June 28, 2017. St. Paul, Minnesota. 11 pages. Interviewed by Sam Aamot.

Coleman, Brandon. "Oral History Interview 1." October 26, 2016. St. Paul, Minnesota. 10 pages.

Coleman, Brandon. "Oral History Interview 2." August 1, 2020. Minneapolis, Minnesota. 5 pages.

Colford, Janie Bining. June 26, 2016. Chanhassen, Minnesota. 21 pages.

DeSanto, Paula. January 26, 2017. Spring Lake Park, Minnesota. 17 pages.

Frank, Kathie Simon. March 15, 2017. Minneapolis, Minnesota. 23 pages.

Frank, Rae Eden. January 31, 2017. Maplewood, Minnesota. 23 pages.

Holman, Deb. May 19, 2017. Duluth, Minnesota. 27 pages.

Holter, Janise. June 14, 2016. St. Paul, Minnesota. 26 pages.

Hooker, Julie. February 2, 2017. St. Paul, Minnesota. 37 pages.

Johnson, Dean. January 20, 2017. Minnetonka, Minnesota. 27 pages.

Levy, Robert. January 13, 2017. Robbinsdale, Minnesota. 32 pages.

Lewis, Lori. June 18, 2016. Oakdale, Minnesota. 25 pages.

McKinney, Rose. June 16, 2016. St. Paul, Minnesota. 23 pages.

Moldenhauer, Richard. March 30, 2017. St. Paul, Minnesota. 17 pages.

O'Neill, Michael. January 19, 2017. Minneapolis, Minnesota. 20 pages.

Perry, Ann. July 6, 2016. Minnetonka, Minnesota. 25 pages.

Perry, Ann. "Trial Discussion." August 16, 2017. Ely, Minnesota. 12 pages.

Powers, Kim. July 5, 2016. Minneapolis, Minnesota. 23 pages.

Purchase, Sue. "Oral History Interview 1." April 27, 2017. Minneapolis, Minnesota. 39 pages.

Purchase, Sue. "Oral History Interview 2." May 9, 2017. Minneapolis, Minnesota. 13 pages.

Purchase, Sue. "Oral History Interview 3." May 30, 2020. Duluth, Minnesota. 11 pages.

Reznikoff, Charles. January 17, 2017. Minneapolis, Minnesota. 22 pages.

Roberts Gyllen, Shelley. August 17, 2017. Ely, Minnesota. 15 pages.

Selleck, Star. June 21, 2016. Minneapolis, Minnesota. 30 pages.

Seppala, Marvin. "Oral History Interview 1." November 6, 2018. Minneapolis, Minnesota. 25 pages.

Seppala, Marvin. "Oral History Interview 2." January 23, 2019. Minneapolis, Minnesota. 41 pages.

Shafie, Yussuf. December 19, 2017. Bloomington, Minnesota. 14 pages.

Tuttle, Andrew. February 16, 2017. Wettingen, Switzerland. 21 pages.

Willenbring, Mark. "Oral History Interview 1." May 17, 2017. St. Paul, Minnesota. 22 pages.

Willenbring, Mark. "Oral History Interview 2." June 14, 2017. St. Paul, Minnesota. 16 pages.

References

Abdi, Cawo Mohamed. "The Newest African-Americans? Somali Struggles for Belonging." In *The Contexts of Diaspora Citizenship: Somali Communities in Finland and the United States*, edited by Päivi Armila, Marko Kananen, and Yasemin Kontkanen, International Perspectives on Migration 17, 19–32. Cham: Springer, 2019. https://doi.org/10.1007/978-3-319-94490-6.

Acker, Caroline Jean, and Sarah W. Tracy. *Altering American Consciousness: The History of Alcohol and Drug Use in the United States, 1800–2000*. Amherst: University of Massachusetts Press, 2004. http://catdir.loc.gov/catdir/toc/ecip045/2003013735.html.

"Alcohol Allowed Here: Minnesota Center Diverges from 12-Step Model." *Alcoholism and Drug Abuse Weekly* 25, no. 13 (2013): 1–1.

Alcoholics Anonymous. "Estimates of A.A. Groups and Members as of December 31, 2020." Revised December 2020. https://www.aa.org/assets/en_us/smf-53_en.pdf.

Alcoholics Anonymous World Services. *Alcoholics Anonymous Big Book*. 2nd ed. Alcoholics Anonymous World Services, 2002.

Alexander, Clinton D., and Brenna Greenfield. "Partnering with Tribal Communities to Promote Well-being and Decrease Opioid Overdose Deaths." Webinar, University of Minnesota, Center for Practice Transformation, July 10, 2020. https://vimeo.com/437234914.

Alexander, Michelle. *The New Jim Crow: Mass Incarceration in the Age of Colorblindness*. New York: New Press, 2012.

American Society of Addiction Medicine. "ASAM Definition of Addiction." Adopted September 15, 2019. https://www.asam.org/Quality-Science/definition-of-addiction.

Amodeo, M. "The Addictive Personality." *Substance Use and Misuse* 50, nos. 8–9 (2015): 1031–36.

Anthony, William A. "A Vision for Psychiatric Rehabilitation Research." *Psychiatric Rehabilitation Journal* 25, no. 1 (2001): 1–2. https://doi.org/10.1037/h0095057.

Anthony, William A., Gregory J. Buell, Sara Sharratt, and Michael E. Althoff. "Efficacy of Psychiatric Rehabilitation." *Psychological Bulletin* 78, no. 6 (1972): 447–56. https://doi.org/10.1037/h0033743.

Anthony, William A., Mikal Cohen, and Marianne Farkas. "The Future of Psychiatric Rehabilitation." *International Journal of Mental Health* 28, no. 1 (1999): 48–68. https://doi.org/10.1080/00207411.1999.11449446.

Ashton, John R., and Howard Seymour. "Public Health and the Origins of the Mersey Model of Harm Reduction." *International Journal of Drug Policy* 21, no. 2 (March 2010): 94–96. https://doi.org/10.1016/j.drugpo.2010.01.004.

Atkinson, Rowland, and John Flint. "Snowball Sampling." In *The SAGE Encyclopedia of Social Science Research Methods*, edited by Michael S. Lewis-Beck, Alan Bryman, and Tim F. Liao, 1044. Thousand Oaks, Calif.: SAGE Publications, 2004. https://doi.org/10.4135/9781412950589.n931.

Aubry, Timothy, and Trysh Travis, eds. *Rethinking Therapeutic Culture*. Chicago: University of Chicago Press, 2015.

Bänziger, Peter-Paul, and Gemma Blok. "'Junkie Kingdoms': Open Drug Scenes and the Narcotic City, Case Study II." Narcotic City: Imaginaries, Practices and Discourses of Public Drug Cultures in European Cities from 1970 until Today. https://narcotic.city/project-research/case-studies/.

Baumgartner, Jesse C., and David C. Radley. "The Spike in Drug Overdose Deaths during the COVID-19 Pandemic and Policy Options to Move Forward." The Commonwealth Fund Blog. March 25, 2021. https://www .commonwealthfund.org/blog/2021/spike-drug-overdose-deaths-during -covid-19-pandemic-and-policy-options-move-forward.

Beattie, Melody Lynn. *Codependent No More: Stop Controlling Others and Start Caring for Yourself.* Center City, Minn.: Hazelden, 1987.

Bebinger, Martha. "Fentanyl-Linked Deaths: The U.S. Opioid Epidemic's Third Wave Begins." *National Public Radio.* March 21, 2019. https://www.npr.org /sections/health-shots/2019/03/21/704557684/fentanyl-linked-deaths -the-u-s-opioid-epidemics-third-wave-begins.

Beck, Jerome. "100 Years of 'Just Say No' Versus 'Just Say Know': Reevaluating Drug Education Goals for the Coming Century." *Evaluation Review* 22, no. 1 (February 1998): 15–45. https://doi.org/10.1177/0193841X9802200102.

Bepko, Claudia, ed. *Feminism and Addiction*. New York: Haworth Press, 1992.

"Big Pharma Buys Clout in Advocacy Over Opioids." *New York Times.* February 8, 2018, B1.

Booth, Martin. *Opium: A History*. New York: St. Martin's Press, 1998.

Boss, Pauline. *Ambiguous Loss: Learning to Live with Unresolved Grief.* Cambridge, Mass.: Harvard University Press, 1999.

Bourgois, Philippe, and Jeff Schonberg. *Righteous Dopefiend.* Berkeley: University of California Press, 2009.

Boyd, Douglas, and Mary Larson, eds. *Oral History and Digital Humanities: Voice, Access, and Engagement.* New York: Palgrave Macmillan, 2014.

Brewer, William. "Overdose Psalm." In *I Know Your Kind: Poems.* Minneapolis: Milkweed Editions, 2017.

Bridge, J. A., S. Iyengar, C. B. Salary, R. P. Barbe, B. Birmaher, H. A. Pincus, L. Ren, and D. A. Brent. "Clinical Response and Risk for Reported Suicidal Ideation and Suicide Attempts in Pediatric Antidepressant Treatment: A

Meta-analysis of Randomized Controlled Trials." JAMA 297, no. 15 (2007): 1683–96.

Bridges, Khiara M. "Race, Pregnancy, and the Opioid Epidemic: White Privilege and the Criminalization of Opioid Use during Pregnancy." *Harvard Law Review* 133, no. 3 (January 2020): 770–851.

Brown, Lyn Mikel, and Carol Gilligan. *Meeting at the Crossroads: Women's Psychology and Girls' Development.* Darby, Penn.: Diane Publishing Company, 1998.

Bumbalo, J. A., and D. E. Young. "The Self-Help Phenomenon." *American Journal of Nursing* 73, no. 9 (1973): 1588–91.

Bury, Judy, Val Morrison, and Sheena McLachlan. *Working with Women and AIDS: Medical, Social and Counselling Issues.* London: Routledge, 2002.

Campbell, Nancy D. *Discovering Addiction: The Science and Politics of Substance Abuse Research.* Ann Arbor: University of Michigan Press, 2007. https://doi.org/10.3998/mpub.269246.

———. *OD: Naloxone and the Politics of Overdose.* Cambridge, Mass: MIT Press, 2020.

———. *Using Women: Gender, Drug Policy, and Social Justice.* New York: Routledge, 2000.

Campbell, Nancy, and Elizabeth Ettorre. *Gendering Addiction: The Politics of Drug Treatment in a Neurochemical World.* New York: Palgrave Macmillan, 2011.

Campbell, Nancy, J. P. Olsen, and Luke Walden. *The Narcotic Farm: The Rise and Fall of America's First Prison for Drug Addicts.* New York: Abrams, 2008.

Cave, Mark, and Stephen M. Sloan, eds. *Listening on the Edge: Oral History in the Aftermath of Crisis.* New York: Oxford University Press, 2014.

Childress, Sarah. "How the Heroin Epidemic Differs in Communities of Color." *Frontline.* PBS. February 23, 2016. https://www.pbs.org/wgbh/frontline/article/how-the-heroin-epidemic-differs-in-communities-of-color/.

Choi, Jiwon. "Maplewood Woman Sentenced to 8 More Years in Opioid Overdose Death." *Minnesota Public Radio.* June 14, 2018. https://www.mprnews.org/story/2018/06/13/beverly-burrell-prosecutors-go-after-dealers-as-opioid-related-deaths-rise.

Clark, Claire D. *The Recovery Revolution: The Battle over Addiction Treatment in the United States.* New York: Columbia University Press, 2017.

Collins, Alexandra B., Jade Boyd, Kanna Hayashi, Hannah L. F. Cooper, Shira Goldenberg, and Ryan McNeil. "Women's Utilization of Housing-Based Overdose Prevention Sites in Vancouver, Canada: An Ethnographic Study." *International Journal of Drug Policy* 76 (February 2020): article 102641. https://doi.org/10.1016/j.drugpo.2019.102641.

Collins, Jon. "It's an Opioid Overdose Death. But Is It a Murder?" *Minnesota Public Radio.* July 27, 2016. https://www.mprnews.org/story/2016/07/27/prosecuting-opioid-overdose-as-murder-heroin-addiction

———. "Son's Overdose Death Drives this Minnesota Legislator's Work."

Minnesota Public Radio News. April 18, 2016. https://www.mprnews.org
/story/2016/04/18/opioid-profiles-dave-baker.

Corkery, Michael, and Katie Thomas. "Drug Industry Wages Opioid Fight Using
an Anti-Addiction Ally." *New York Times.* February 8, 2018. https://www
.nytimes.com/2018/02/08/business/opioids-addiction-pharma.html.

Courtwright, David. *The Age of Addiction: How Bad Habits Became Big Business.* Cambridge, Mass.: Belknap Press of Harvard University Press, 2019.

———. *Dark Paradise: Opiate Addiction in America before 1940.* Cambridge,
Mass.: Harvard University Press, 1982.

———. *Forces of Habit: Drugs and the Making of the Modern World.* Cambridge,
Mass.: Harvard University Press, 2002.

———. "The Prepared Mind: Marie Nyswander, Methadone Maintenance,
and the Metabolic Theory of Addiction." *Addiction* 92, no. 3 (March 1997):
257–65.

Courtwright, David T., Herman Joseph, and Don Des Jarlais. *Addicts Who
Survived: An Oral History of Narcotic Use in America before 1965.* Knoxville:
University of Tennessee Press, 2013.

Creedon, Timothy B., and Benjamin Lê Cook. "Access to Mental Health Care
Increased but Not for Substance Use, While Disparities Remain." *Health
Affairs* 35, no. 6 (2016): 1017–21. http://doi.org/10.1377/hlthaff.2016.0098.

Crosby, Jackie. "Obituary: Toni St. Pierre Blazed Trail for Girls' Sports." *Star
Tribune.* February 16, 2013. https://www.startribune.com/obituary-toni
-st-pierre-blazed-trail-for-girls-sports/191555011/.

DeLaquil, M., S. Giesel, and N. Wright. "Preliminary 2020 Drug Overdose
Deaths." Minnesota Department of Health. April 27, 2021. https://www
.health.state.mn.us/communities/opioids/documents
/drugoverdosereport2020.pdf.

DeSanto, Paula. *Effective Addiction Treatment: The Minnesota Alternative.*
Spring Lake Park: Minnesota Alternatives LLC, 2012.

Des Jarlais, Don C. "Harm Reduction in the USA: The Research Perspective
and an Archive to David Purchase." *Harm Reduction Journal* 14, no. 1 (26
2017): 51. https://doi.org/10.1186/s12954-017-0178-6.

Des Jarlais, Don C., Courtney McKnight, Cullen Goldblatt, and David Purchase. "Doing Harm Reduction Better: Syringe Exchange in the United
States." *Addiction* 104, no. 9 (September 2009): 1441–46. https://doi.org
/10.1111/j.1360-0443.2008.02465.x.

Des Jarlais, Don C., Courtney McKnight, and Judith Milliken. "Public Funding
of US Syringe Exchange Programs." *Journal of Urban Health: Bulletin of the
New York Academy of Medicine* 81, no. 1 (March 2004): 118–21. https://doi
.org/10.1093/jurban/jth093.

Des Jarlais, Don C., Denise Paone, Samuel R Friedman, Nina Peyser, and
Robert G Newman. "Regulating Controversial Programs for Unpopular
People: Methadone Maintenance and Syringe Exchange Programs." *Ameri-
can Journal of Public Health* 85, no. 11 (1995): 1577–84.

Diaz, Lucy. "Student Saves Life with Naloxone Drug from Macalester History
Class." *The Mac Weekly.* December 10, 2020. https://themacweekly.com

/79320/features/student-saves-life-with-naloxone-drug-from-macalester
-history-class/.

Doepke, Matthias, and Fabrizio Zilibotti. *Love, Money, and Parenting: How Economics Explains the Way We Raise Our Kids*. Princeton, N.J.: Princeton University Press, 2019.

Duwe, Grant. "Prison-Based Chemical Dependency Treatment in Minnesota: An Outcome Evaluation." *Journal of Experimental Criminology* 6, no. 1 (March 2010): 57–81. https://www.ojp.gov/ncjrs/virtual-library/abstracts /prison-based-chemical-dependency-treatment-minnesota-outcome.

Dwyer, Colin. "Your Guide to the Massive (and Massively Complex) Opioid Litigation." *National Public Radio*. October 15, 2019. https://www.npr.org /sections/health-shots/2019/10/15/761537367/your-guide-to-the-massive -and-massively-complex-opioid-litigation.

Earnshaw, Valerie, Laramie Smith, and Michael Copenhaver. "Drug Addiction Stigma in the Context of Methadone Maintenance Therapy: An Investigation into Understudied Sources of Stigma." *International Journal of Mental Health and Addiction* 11, no. 1 (2013): 110–22.

Edwards, Bob. "Needle Exchange." *Morning Edition, National Public Radio*. April 21, 1998. https://www.npr.org/templates/story/story.php?storyId =1026318.

Erickson, Patricia, Diane Riley, Yuet Cheung, and Patrick O'Hare, eds. *Harm Reduction: A New Practice for Drug Policies and Programs*. Toronto: University of Toronto Press, 1997.

Farrugia, Adrian, Suzanne Fraser, Robyn Dwyer, Renae Fomiatti, Joanne Neale, Paul Dietze, and John Strang. "Take-Home Naloxone and the Politics of Care." *Sociology of Health and Illness* 41, no. 2 (2019): 427–43. https:// doi.org/10.1111/1467-9566.12848.

Fletcher, Anne. *Inside Rehab: The Surprising Truth about Addiction Treatment—and How to Get Help That Works*. New York: Viking Press, 2013.

Foote, Susan Bartlett. *The Crusade for Forgotten Souls: Reforming Minnesota's Mental Institutions, 1946–1954*. Minneapolis: University of Minnesota Press, 2018.

Frisch, John. "Our Years in Hell: American Addicts Tell Their Story, 1829–1914." *Journal of Psychedelic Drugs* 9, no. 3 (September 1977): 199–208.

Frydl, Kathleen. *The Drug Wars in America, 1940–1973*. Cambridge: Cambridge University Press, 2013.

Frye, Marilyn. *The Politics of Reality: Essays in Feminist Theory*. Crossing Press Feminist Series. Trumansburg, N.Y.: Crossing Press, 1983.

Garrett, Roberta. *We Need to Talk about Family: Essays on Neoliberalism, the Family, and Popular Culture*. Newcastle-upon-Tyne: Cambridge Scholars Publishing, 2016.

Gavin, Kara. "UMHS, Addiction Community Mourn Death of Patrick Gibbons." *The University Record*. University of Michigan. March 31, 2014. https:// record.umich.edu/articles/umhs-addiction-community-mourns-death -patrick-gibbons/.

Giesel, S., M. DeLaquil, and N. Wright. "Drug Overdose Deaths among Minnesota Residents from January through June 2020." Minnesota Department of Health. December 2, 2020. https://www.health.state.mn.us/communities /opioids/documents/drugoverdosescovid.pdf.

Gilligan, Carol. *In a Different Voice.* Cambridge, Mass.: Harvard University Press, 2009.

Glasner-Edwards, Suzette. *The Addiction Recovery Skills Workbook: Changing Addictive Behaviors Using CBT, Mindfulness, and Motivational Interviewing Techniques.* Oakland, Calif.: New Harbinger Publications, 2015.

Gowan, Teresa, and Sarah Whetstone. "Making the Criminal Addict: Subjectivity and Social Control in a Strong-Arm Rehab." *Punishment and Society* 14 (January 13, 2012): 69–93. https://doi.org/10.1177/1462474511424684.

Greenfield, Brenna. "Opioid Overdose Fatality Reviews: Finding New Opportunities for Healing and Prevention." National Institute on Drug Abuse, Subaward from National Drug Early Warning System, 2019.

Grim, Ryan. "Minnesota State Senator Chris Eaton to Push Legislation to Reform Heroin Treatment." *The Huffington Post.* February 2, 2015. https:// www.huffpost.com/entry/heroin-treatment_n_6598876.

Gunderson, Dan. "'How Can We Prevent the Heart from Breaking?' White Earth Reviews Opioid Overdose Deaths." *Minnesota Public Radio.* December 18, 2019. https://www.mprnews.org/story/2019/12/18/how-can-we-prevent -the-heart-from-breaking-review-of-white-earth-opioid-overdose-deaths.

Hamilton, Paula, and Linda Shopes, eds. *Oral History and Public Memories.* Philadelphia: Temple University Press, 2008.

Hart, Carl L. *High Price: A Neuroscientist's Journey of Self-Discovery That Challenges Everything You Know about Drugs and Society.* New York: Harper Perennial, 2014.

Harvey, Gary. "Dance at Apple Valley Will Cap Drug Awareness Campaign." *Star Tribune.* October 26, 1989: 01Y.

Heikkila, Kim. "'Everybody Thinks It's Right to Give the Child Away': Unwed Mothers at Booth Memorial Hospital, 1961–63." *Minnesota History* 65, no. 6 (2017): 229–41.

Helmstetter, Craig. "Racial Disparities in Minnesota: Better, Worse, or the Same?" *Minnesota Compass.* August 16, 2016. https://www.mncompass.org /trends/insights/2016-08-16-disparities-trends.

Henderson, Elizabeth Connell. *Understanding Addiction.* Jackson: University Press of Mississippi, 2009.

Hertel, Lee. Harm Reduction History Harvest Transcript. Available from *Women with a Point!* and *Access Works,* https://amycsullivan.net/wap/items/show /83.

Hevesi, Dennis. "Dave Purchase Dies at 73; Led Early Needle Exchange." *New York Times.* January 27, 2013. https://www.nytimes.com/2013/01/28/us /dave-purchase-who-led-needle-exchange-movement-dies-at-73.html.

Hoffman, Marella. *Practicing Oral History to Improve Public Policies and Programs.* New York: Routledge, 2018.

Horvath, A. Thomas. "Smart Recovery®: Addiction Recovery Support from a Cognitive-Behavioral Perspective." *Journal of Rational-Emotive and Cognitive-Behavior Therapy* 18, no. 3 (2000): 181–91.

Huddleston, C. West, Douglas B. Marlowe, and Rachel Casebolt. "Painting the Current Picture: A National Report Card on Drug Courts and Other Problem-Solving Court Programs in the United States." National Drug Court Institute. May 2008. https://www.ndci.org/sites/default/files /ndci/PCPII1_web%5B1%5D.pdf.

Ibrahim, Hudda O. *From Somalia to Snow: How Central Minnesota Became Home to Somalis.* Edina, Minn.: Beaver's Pond Press, 2017.

Ibrahim, Mukhtar M. "'Monster in Our Community': East African Youth Break the Silence over Addiction." *Minnesota Public Radio.* October 30, 2019. https:// www.mprnews.org/story/2019/10/30/monster-in-our-community-east -african-youth-break-the-silence-over-addiction.

Irvine, Leslie J. "Codependency and Recovery: Gender, Self, and Emotions in Popular Self-Help." *Symbolic Interaction* 18, no. 2 (1995): 145–63. https:// doi.org/10.1525/si.1995.18.2.145.

Jack, Jordynn. *Autism and Gender: From Refrigerator Mothers to Computer Geeks.* Urbana: University of Illinois Press, 2014. https://www.jstor.org /stable/10.5406/j.ctt7zw5k5.5.

James, Keturah, and Ayana Jordan. "The Opioid Crisis in Black Communities." *Journal of Law, Medicine, and Ethics* 46, no. 2 (2018): 404–21.

Jarmolowicz, D. P., E. T. Mueller, M. N. Koffarnus, A. E. Carter, K. M. Gatchalian, and W. K. Bickel. "Executive Dysfunction in Addiction." In *The Wiley-Blackwell Handbook of Addiction Psychopharmacology,* edited by J. MacKillop and H. de Wit. Hoboken, New Jersey: Wiley-Blackwell, 2013.

Jason, Leonard A., Joseph R. Ferrari, and Margaret Davis. *Creating Communities for Addiction Recovery: The Oxford House Model.* Hoboken: Taylor and Francis, 2014.

Karlen, Neal. "Greetings from Minnesober." *New York Times.* May 28, 1995.

Keilman, John. "Dan Bigg Remembered as 'Revolutionary' for Approach to Heroin Crisis, Pioneered Life-Saving Naloxone, Needle Handouts." *Chicago Tribune,* August 22, 2018.

Kelly, Peter J., Dayle Raftery, Frank P. Deane, Amanda L. Baker, David Hunt, and Anthony Shakeshaft. "From Both Sides: Participant and Facilitator Perceptions of SMART Recovery Groups." *Drug and Alcohol Review* 36, no. 3 (2017): 325–32. https://doi.org/10.1111/dar.12416.

Kersten, Katherine. "Dare to Ask Whether D.A.R.E. Is Doing Kids More Harm than Good." *Star Tribune.* September 17, 1997: 17A.

Klein, A. A., and M. D. Seppala. "Medication-Assisted Treatment for Opioid Use Disorder within a 12-Step Based Treatment Center: Feasibility and Initial Results." *Journal of Substance Abuse Treatment* 104 (September 2019): 51–63.

Knowlton, Judith M., and Rebecca D. Chaitin. *Detachment and Enabling.* Minneapolis: Hazelden Publishing, 2010.

Knudsen, Hannah, et al. "Service Delivery and Use of Evidence-Based Treatment Practices in Adolescent Substance Abuse Treatment Settings."

Project Report, 2008, Robert Wood Johnson Foundation, Substance Abuse Policy Research.

Koumpilova, Mila. "Somali Social Worker Opens Substance Abuse Treatment Center Aimed at African Refugees." *Star Tribune.* June 3, 2015.

Krestan, Jo-Ann, and Claudia Bepko. "Codependency: The Social Reconstruction of Female Experience." In *Feminism and Addiction,* edited by Claudia Bepko, 49–66. New York: Haworth Press, 1992.

Kuhn, Cynthia, Scott Swartzwelder, Wilkie Wilson, Leigh Heather Wilson, and Jeremy Foster. *Buzzed: The Straight Facts about the Most Used and Abused Drugs from Alcohol to Ecstasy.* 4th ed. New York: W. W. Norton, 2014.

LaSalle, Lindsay. "An Overdose Death Is Not Murder: Why Drug-Induced Homicide Laws Are Counterproductive and Inhumane." Drug Policy Alliance, November 2017. https://drugpolicy.org/sites/default/files/dpa _drug_induced_homicide_report_0.pdf.

Lerner, Barron. *One for the Road: Drunk Driving since 1990.* Baltimore, Md.: Johns Hopkins University Press, 2011.

Levine, Noah. *Refuge Recovery: A Buddhist Path to Recovering from Addiction.* San Francisco: HarperOne, 2014.

Levine, Susan. *School Lunch Politics: The Surprising History of America's Favorite Welfare Program.* Politics and Society in Twentieth-Century America. Princeton, N.J.: Princeton University Press, 2008.

Lippold, Kumiko M., Christopher M. Jones, Emily O'Malley Olsen, and Brett P. Giroir. "Racial/Ethnic and Age Group Differences in Opioid and Synthetic Opioid-Involved Overdose Deaths among Adults Aged ≥18 Years in Metropolitan Areas—United States, 2015–2017." *Morbidity and Mortality Weekly Report* 68 (2019): 967–73. https://doi.org/10.15585/mmwr.mm6843a3.

Lisansky Gomberg, Edith S. "On Terms Used and Abused: The Concept of 'Codependency.'" *Drugs and Society* 3, nos. 3–4 (November 22, 1989): 113–32. https://doi.org/10.1300/J023v03n03_05.

Marnati, Raeanna. "Wetterling Family Speaks Out on Arrest of 'Person of Interest.'" FOX21 Local News. November 3, 2015. https://www.fox21online .com/2015/11/03/wetterling-family-speaks-out-on-arrest-of-person-of -interest/.

Mars, Sarah G., Philippe Bourgois, George Karandinos, Fernando Montero, and Daniel Ciccarone. "'Every "Never" I Ever Said Came True': Transitions from Opioid Pills to Heroin Injecting." *International Journal of Drug Policy* 25, no. 2 (March 2014): 257–266.

Maté, Gabor. *In the Realm of Hungry Ghosts: Close Encounters with Addiction.* Lyons, Colo.: Ergos Institute; Berkeley: North Atlantic Books, 2008.

Maynes, Mary Jo, Jennifer Pierce, and Barbara Laslett. *Telling Stories: The Use of Personal Narratives in the Social Sciences and History.* Ithaca, N.Y.: Cornell University Press, 2008.

McKeever, Patricia, and Karen-Lee Miller. "Mothering Children Who Have Disabilities: A Bourdieusian Interpretation of Maternal Practices." *Social Science and Medicine* 59, no. 6 (2004): 1177–91.

Menakem, Resmaa. *My Grandmother's Hands: Racialized Trauma and the*

Pathway to Mending Our Hearts and Bodies. Las Vegas: Central Recovery Press, 2017.

Meyers, Robert J., William R. Miller, Dina E. Hill, and J. Scott Tonigan. "Community Reinforcement and Family Training (CRAFT): Engaging Unmotivated Drug Users in Treatment." *Journal of Substance Abuse* 10, no. 3 (1998): 291–308.

Midwest Center for Trauma and Emotional Healing. "Adaptive Internal Relational (AIR) Network Model: An Overview." Copyright 2015 McClelland, Miller and Solon. https://www.mwtraumacenter.com/adaptive-internal-relational-model-overv.

Miller, Kay, and Staff Writer. "How Melody Beattie Became 'codependent no more.'" *Star Tribune* [METRO Edition]. August 7, 1988.

Minnesota Board of Pharmacy. "Minnesota Prescription Monitoring Program." Accessed July 30, 2020. https://www.pmp.pharmacy.state.mn.us/.

Minnesota Compass. "Somali Population." http://www.mncompass.org/demographics/cultural-communities/somali.

Minnesota Department of Corrections. "Fact Sheet: Substance Use Disorder Treatment Services in Prison." December 2019. https://mn.gov/doc/assets/Substance%20Use%20Disorder%20Treatment_tcm1089-413914.pdf.

———. "Minnesota Sentencing Guidelines and Commentary." August 1, 2016. https://mn.gov/msgc-stat/documents/2016%20Guidelines/11_17_2016_Update_August2016_Guidelines.pdf.

Minnesota Department of Employment and Economic Development. "Racial Disparities." Accessed August 2, 2020. https://mn.gov/deed/data/lmi-reports/racial-disparities/

Minnesota Department of Health. "HIV Outbreak Response and Case Counts." March 31, 2021. https://www.health.state.mn.us/diseases/hiv/stats/hiv.html#cases1.

———. "Opioids: Drug Overdose Dashboard." July 17, 2020. https://www.health.state.mn.us/opioiddashboard.

———. "Preliminary 2019 Drug Overdose Deaths: A Return to the State's Overall Trend." 2019. https://www.health.state.mn.us/communities/opioids/documents/2019prelimdeathreport.pdf.

Minnesota Department of Human Services. "Alcohol, Drug, and Other Addictions: Policies and Procedures." Updated November 22, 2016. https://mn.gov/dhs/partners-and-providers/policies-procedures/alcohol-drug-other-addictions/.

Minnesota Department of Human Services. "GRH [Group Residential Housing] Basis—Drug/Alcohol Addiction." https://www.dhs.state.mn.us/main/idcplg?IdcService=GET_DYNAMIC_CONVERSION&RevisionSelectionMethod=LatestReleased&dDocName=cm_00131836#.

———. "Minnesota State Targeted Response to the Opioid Crisis: Project Narrative." April 19, 2017. https://mn.gov/dhs/assets/mn-opioid-str-project-narrative-april-2017_tcm1053-289624.pdf.

Monico, Laura B., Jan Gryczynski, Shannon Gwin Mitchell, Robert P. Schwartz, Kevin E. O'Grady, and Jerome H. Jaffe. "Buprenorphine Treatment and

12-Step Meeting Attendance: Conflicts, Compatibilities, and Patient Outcomes." *Journal of Substance Abuse Treatment* 57 (October 2015): 89–95. https://doi.org/10.1016/j.jsat.2015.05.005.

Morain, Claudia. "Needle Exchange Programs Can Prevent AIDS." In *AIDS: Opposing Viewpoints*, edited by Michael D. Biskup and Karin Swisher, Opposing Viewpoints Series, 130–35. San Diego, Calif.: Greenhaven Press, 1992.

MPR News. "Beverly Burrell Delivers a Statement and Is Sentenced." YouTube. September 28, 2017. https://youtu.be/zEaj1gNXKmw.

Mullen, Mike. "Read Victim Impact Letters about Twin Cities Heroin Dealer Beverly Burrell." *City Pages*. October 11, 2017. https://www.mnhs.org /newspapers/hub/city-pages.

Murakawa, Naomi. "Toothless: The Methamphetamine 'Epidemic,' 'Meth Mouth,' and the Racial Construction of Drug Scares." *Du Bois Review: Social Science Research on Race* 8, no. 1 (2011): 219–28. https://doi.org /10.1017/S1742058X11000208.

Murphy, Esme. "Lawmakers Chris Eaton, Dave Baker Talk Opioids after Personal Losses." WCCO Sunday Morning. February 18, 2018. https:// minnesota.cbslocal.com/video/3812792-lawmakers-chris-eaton-dave -baker-talk-opioids-after-personal-losses/.

Musto, David. *The American Disease: Origins of Narcotic Control.* 3rd ed. Oxford: Oxford University Press, 1999.

Nakken, Jane. *Enabling Change: When Your Child Returns Home from Treatment.* Center City, Minn.: Hazelden Foundation, 1985.

———. "Issues in Adolescent Chemical Dependency Assessment." *Journal of Adolescent Chemical Dependency* 1, no. 3 (1991): 77–99.

Nar-Anon Family Group. *Sharing Experience, Strength, and Hope.* 2nd ed. Torrance, Calif.: Nar-Anon Family Group Conference Approved Literature, 2007.

Narcotics Anonymous. "Regarding Methadone and Other Drug Replacement Programs." World Service Board of Trustees Bulletin #29. 1996. https:// www.na.org/?ID=bulletins-bull29.

National Council on Alcohol and Drug Addiction. "That's How." January 29, 2015. https://youtu.be/nPF-Juks2N0.

———. "All American Girl—Heroin Super Bowl Commercial." February 3, 2016. https://youtu.be/P-i6PlKdMug.

National Institute on Drug Abuse. "Opioid Overdose Crisis." March 11, 2021. https://www.drugabuse.gov/drug-topics/opioids/opioid-overdose-crisis.

"Needle Exchange for Addicts Wins Foothold against AIDS in Tacoma." *New York Times.* January 23, 1989.

Nelson, Margaret K. *Parenting Out of Control: Anxious Parents in Uncertain Times.* New York: New York University Press, 2010.

Netherland, Julie, and Helena B. Hansen. "The War on Drugs that Wasn't: Wasted Whiteness, 'Dirty Doctors,' and Race in Media Coverage of Prescription Opioid Misuse." *Culture, Medicine, and Psychiatry* 40, no. 4 (2016): 664–86. https://doi.org/10.1007/s11013-016-9496-5.

———. "White Opioids: Pharmaceutical Race and the War on Drugs that Wasn't."

BioSocieties 12, no. 2 (June 2017): 217–38. https://doi.org/10.1057/biosoc .2015.46.

Neutkens, Debra. "Journey with Pain Pills Often Dead End with Heroin." *White Bear Press.* Last updated January 8, 2015. https://www.presspubs .com/white_bear/news/journey-with-pain-pills-often-dead-end-with -heroin/article_9b43adaa-907a-11e4-a6ee-63e8b6c082bf.html.

Newcombe, Russell, and Allan Parry. "The Mersey Harm-Reduction Model: A Strategy for Dealing with Drug Users." Presentation at the International Conference on Drug Policy Reform, Bethesda, Maryland, October 22, 1988.

niin gikenjige Harm Reduction Coalition. "The 8th Annual Harm Reduction Summit." April 29, 2019 – May 3, 2019. Last updated April 5, 2019. https:// www.evensi.us/8th-annual-harm-reduction-summit-shooting-star -casino/301274201.

Nixon, Sara Jo. "Executive Functioning among Young People in Relation to Alcohol Use." *Current Opinion in Psychiatry* 26, no. 4 (2013): 305–9.

Novotny, Gary A., Niki U. Cotton-Oldenburg, Bill Bond, and Bob Tracy. "The Minnesota Pharmacy Syringe Access Initiative: A Successful Statewide Program to Increase Injection Drug User Access to Sterile Syringes." *Journal of the American Pharmaceutical Association* 42, no. 6, Suppl. 2 (November–December 2002): S21–22. https://doi.org/10.1331/1086-5802 .42.0.s21.novotny.

Nowinski, J. *The Twelve Step Facilitation Outpatient Program.* Center City, Minn.: Hazelden, 2006.

Nowinski, J., and S. Baker. *The Twelve Step Facilitation Handbook: A Guide to Recovery from Chemical Dependence.* 2nd ed. Center City, Minn.: Hazelden, 2003.

Nowinski, J., S. Baker, and L. Carroll. *The Twelve Step Facilitation Therapy Manual: A Clinical Research Guide for Therapists Treating Individuals with Alcohol Abuse and Dependence.* Project MATCH Monograph Series 1. Rockville, Md.: National Institute on Alcohol Abuse and Alcoholism, 1992.

Obermeyer, Chad. "Prozac and the Great U-Turn in American Psychiatry." PhD diss., Harvard University, 2001.

Oral History Association. "OHA Principles and Best Practices." Adopted October 2018. https://www.oralhistory.org/principles-and-best-practices -revised-2018/.

Orenstein, Peggy. *Schoolgirls: Young Women, Self Esteem, and the Confidence Gap.* New York: Knopf Doubleday, 2013.

O'Connor, Patrick G., Robert J. Sokol, and Gail D'Onofrio. "Addiction Medicine: The Birth of a New Discipline." JAMA *Internal Medicine* 174, no. 11 (2014): 1717–18.

O'Hare, P. A. *The Reduction of Drug-Related Harm.* London: Routledge, 1992.

O'Hare, Pat. "Merseyside, the First Harm Reduction Conferences, and the Early History of Harm Reduction." *International Journal of Drug Policy* 18, no. 2 (March 2007): 141–44. https://doi.org/10.1016/j.drugpo.2007.01.003.

Palombi, Laura C., and Cynthia P. Koh-Knox. "The Drug Court Pharmacist: Expanding Pharmacy Practice and Addressing Substance Abuse."

INNOVATIONS in Pharmacy 7, no. 3 (October 11, 2016). https://doi.org /10.24926/iip.v7i3.455.

Parekh, Ranna, and Ed W. Childs, eds. Stigma and Prejudice: Touchstones in Understanding Diversity in Healthcare. Cham: Springer International Publishing, 2016.

Paris, Francesca. "Militia Members Plead Guilty to 2017 Minnesota Mosque Bombing." National Public Radio. January 24, 2019. https://www.npr.org /2019/01/24/688402478/militia-members-plead-guilty-to-2017-minnesota -mosque-bombing.

Pipher, Mary Bray. Reviving Ophelia: Saving the Selves of Adolescent Girls. New York: Putnam, 1994.

Planalp, Colin, Robert Hest, and Megan Lahr. "The Opioid Epidemic: National Trends in Opioid-Related Overdose Deaths from 2000 to 2017." State Health Access Data Assistance Center. June 2019. https://www.shadac.org/sites /default/files/publications/2019%20NATIONAL%20opioid%20brief %20FINAL%20VERSION.pdf.

Plummer Lee, ChienTi, Troy Beckert, and Ian Marsee. "Well-Being and Substance Use in Emerging Adulthood: The Role of Individual and Family Factors in Childhood and Adolescence." Journal of Child and Family Studies 27, no. 12 (December 2018): 3853–65. https://doi.org/10.1007/s10826-018-1227-9.

"Pride Still Stands Out as Site Tailored to LGBT Clients." Alcoholism and Drug Abuse Weekly 24, no. 22 (June 4, 2012): 1–1.

"Public Opinion Poll Shows Deep-Seated Conflict about Addiction as a Disease." Alcoholism and Drug Abuse Weekly 18, no. 33 (August 21, 2006): 1–4.

Quinones, Sam. Dreamland: The True Tale of America's Opiate Epidemic. New York: Bloomsbury Publishing, 2015.

Raskin, Nathaniel J. Contributions to Client-Centered Therapy and the Person-Centered Approach. Person-Centred Approach and Client-Centred Therapy Essential Readers. Ross-on-Wye: PCCS, 2004.

Reagan, Nancy. "Just Say No." School Safety, Spring 1986, 4–5.

Reed, Kayla, James M. Duncan, Mallory Lucier-Greer, Courtney Fixelle, and Anthony J. Ferraro. "Helicopter Parenting and Emerging Adult Self-Efficacy: Implications for Mental and Physical Health." Journal of Child and Family Studies 25, no. 10 (October 2016): 3136–49. https://doi.org/10.1007 /s10826-016-0466-x.

Riley, Diane, and Pat O'Hare. "Harm Reduction: History, Definition, and Practice." In Harm Reduction: National and International Perspectives, edited by James A. Inciardi and Lana D. Harrison, 1–26. Thousand Oaks: SAGE Publications, 2000. https://doi.org/10.4135/9781452220680.

Roble, Abdi, and Douglas F. Rutledge. The Somali Diaspora: A Journey Away. Minneapolis: University of Minnesota Press, 2008.

Rogers, Carl R. Client-Centered Therapy: Its Current Practice, Implications, and Theory. Houghton Mifflin Psychological Series. Boston: Houghton Mifflin, 1951.

Rosenblum, Gail. "'Good Samaritan' Law Essential for Drug Antidote to Succeed." Star Tribune. March 10, 2014. https://www.startribune.com

/rosenblum-good-samaritan-law-essential-for-drug-antidote-to-succeed
/249364871/.

Rotskoff, Lori E. *Love on the Rocks: Men, Women, and Alcohol in Post–World War II America.* Chapel Hill: University of North Carolina Press, 2002.

———. "Sober Husbands and Supportive Wives: Marital Dramas of Alcoholism in Post–World War II America." In *Altering American Consciousness: The History of Alcohol and Drug Use in the United States, 1800–2000,* edited by Sarah W. Tracy and Caroline Jean Acker, 298–326. Amherst: University of Massachusetts Press, 2004

Savary, Jean-Félix, Chris Hallam, and Dave Bewley-Taylor. "The Swiss Four Pillars Policy: An Evolution From Local Experimentation to Federal Law." The Beckley Foundation Drug Policy Programme. May 2009.

Schach, Jean Marie. "Impact of Nar-Anon Family Support Group upon Family Members of Heroin Addicts." MSW thesis, California State University, Sacramento, 1987.

Schwartz, Jason. "A Terrible Loss for Dawn Farm and the Field." *Addiction and Recovery News* (blog). March 27, 2014. https://addictionandrecoverynews .wordpress.com/2014/03/27/a-terrible-loss-for-dawn-farm-and-the-field/.

Seth, P., L. Scholl, R. A. Rudd, and S. Bacon. "Overdose Deaths Involving Opioids, Cocaine, and Psychostimulants—United States, 2015–2016." *Morbidity and Mortality Weekly Report* 67 (2018): 349–58.

Sharpless, Rebecca. "The History of Oral History." In *History of Oral History: Foundations and Methodology,* edited by Thomas L. Charlton, Lois E. Myers, and Rebecca Sharpless, 9–32. Lanham, Md.: Altamira Press, 2007.

Sheff, David. *Clean: Overcoming Addiction and Ending America's Greatest Tragedy.* New York: Eamon Dolan, 2013.

Shorter, Edward. *A History of Psychiatry: From the Era of the Asylum to the Age of Prozac.* New York: Wiley, 1998.

Shullenberger, Bonnie. "Needle Exchange Programs Will Not Prevent AIDS." In *AIDS: Opposing Viewpoints,* edited by Michael D. Biskup and Karin Swisher, Opposing Viewpoints Series. San Diego, Calif.: Greenhaven Press, 1992.

Siegel, Zachary. "Why Activists Think the Super Bowl's Heroin PSA Is Stigmatizing." The Fix. February 8, 2016. https://www.thefix.com/ why-activists-think-super-bowl%E2%80%99s-heroin-psa-stigmatizing.

Singh, Ilina. "Doing Their Jobs: Mothering with Ritalin in a Culture of Mother-Blame." *Social Science and Medicine* 59, no. 6 (2004): 1193–1205.

Slater, Lauren. *The Drugs That Changed Our Minds: The History of Psychiatry in Ten Treatments.* London: Simon and Schuster, 2018.

Smith, Mary Lynn. "Three Heroin Deaths, One Dealer: 'She Sold It to Them Knowing It Was Bad.'" *Star Tribune.* July 21, 2016. https://www.startribune .com/july-21-2016-3-heroin-deaths-1-dealer-she-sold-it-to-them-knowing -it-was-bad/387680791/.

———. "Twin Cities Heroin Dealer Gets 14 Years for Overdose Deaths of Two Men." *Star Tribune.* September 29, 2017. https://www.startribune.com

/twin-cities-heroin-drug-dealer-to-be-sentenced-thursday-for-two-fatal
-overdoses/448456643/.

Solon, Phylis, and Gabor Maté. "The Biology of Loss: A Trauma-Informed
Perspective on Treating Addiction and Concurrent Disorders." January 27,
2017. Seminar at Coffman Memorial Union, University of Minnesota.

Somali TV Minnesota. "The Stigma of Substance Abuse for Women, by Biftu
[Jillo]." YouTube. October 27, 2019. https://youtu.be/idUuPeeTBik.

Spencer, Merianne, Margaret Warner, and Brigham Bastian. "Drug Overdose
Deaths Involving Fentanyl, 2011–2016." *National Vital Statistics Reports* 68,
no. 3 (March 21, 2019): 19.

Spicer, Jerry. *The Minnesota Model: The Evolution of the Multidisciplinary
Approach to Addiction Recovery.* Center City, Minn.: Hazelden Educational
Materials, 1993.

Spindler, Amy M. "The 90's Version of the Decadent Look." *New York Times.*
Style section. May 7, 1996. https://www.nytimes.com/1996/05/07/style
/the-90-s-version-of-the-decadent-look.html.

Springer, Edith. "Effective AIDS Prevention with Active Drug Users: The Harm
Reduction Model." *Journal of Chemical Dependency Treatment* 4, no. 2
(1992): 141–57.

———. "Worker Stances for Clients Who Use Drugs." Handout, 1996. Women
with a Point! and Access Works archive. https://amycsullivan.net/wap
/items/show/38.

Substance Abuse and Mental Health Services Administration. "Buprenorphine."
Last updated March 12, 2021. https://www.samhsa.gov/medication
-assisted-treatment/treatment/buprenorphine.

———. "Naloxone." Last updated August 19, 2020. https://www.samhsa.gov
/medication-assisted-treatment/treatment/naloxone.

———. "National Survey of Substance Abuse Treatment Services (N-SSATS):
2019, Data on Substance Abuse Treatment Facilities." August 20, 2020.
https://www.samhsa.gov/data/report/national-survey-substance-abuse
-treatment-services-n-ssats-2019-data-substance-abuse.

———. "Not Your Mother's Scare Tactics: The Changing Landscape of Fear-
Based Messaging Research." Rhode Island Prevention Resource Center.
https://www.riprc.org/wp-content/uploads/2016/10/The-Changing
-Landscape-of-Fear-based-Messaging-Research_10.7.16.pdf.

———. "Medications for Opioid Use Disorder – Executive Summary." Treatment Improvement Protocol (TIP) 63. May 2020. https://store.samhsa
.gov/product/TIP-63-Medications-for-Opioid-Use-Disorder-Executive
-Summary/PEP20-02-01-005.

Sullivan, Amy C. "'What Fear Is Like': The Legacy of Trauma, Safety, and
Security after the 1977 Girl Scout Murders." PhD diss., University of Illinois
at Chicago, 2013. https://hdl.handle.net/10027/10039.

Swerdlow, Amy. *Women Strike for Peace: Traditional Motherhood and Radical
Politics in the 1960s.* Women in Culture and Society. Chicago: University of
Chicago Press, 1993.

Tracy, Sarah W., and Caroline Jean Acker, eds. *Altering American Consciousness:*

The History of Alcohol and Drug Use in the United States, 1800–2000.
Amherst: University of Massachusetts Press, 2004.

Travis, Trysh. "The Intersectional Origins of Women's 'Substance Abuse' Treatment: Learning from Detroit's Woman Center, 1970–1985." *Contemporary Drug Problems* 44, no. 4 (2017): 265–85.

———. *The Language of the Heart: A Cultural History of the Recovery Moment from Alcoholics Anonymous to Oprah Winfrey.* Chapel Hill: University of North Carolina Press, 2009.

U.S. Census Bureau. "QuickFacts: Minnesota; United States." Accessed July 30, 2020. https://www.census.gov/quickfacts/fact/table/MN,US/RHI325219.

U.S. Centers for Disease Control and Prevention. "Understanding the Epidemic | Opioid Basics | Opioid Overdose | Injury Center." March 17, 2021. https://www.cdc.gov/drugoverdose/epidemic/index.html.

U.S. Food and Drug Administration. "Timeline of Selected FDA Activities and Significant Events Addressing Opioid Misuse and Abuse." Accessed December 2017. https://www.fda.gov/media/120265/download.

———. "Vivitrol Drug Facts and Label." Revised October 2010. https://www.accessdata.fda.gov/drugsatfda_docs/label/2010/021897s015lbl.pdf

U.S. National Library of Medicine. "Current Trends in the Therapy for Narcotic Addiction." Digital Collections. 29 minutes. Accessed June 25, 2020. https://collections.nlm.nih.gov/catalog/nlm:nlmuid-8600251A-vid.

Vandenberg-Daves, Jodi. *Modern Motherhood: An American History.* New Brunswick, N.J.: Rutgers University Press, 2014. https://www.jstor.org/stable/j.ctt6wqb20.3.

Wailoo, Keith. *Pain: A Political History.* Baltimore, Md.: Johns Hopkins University Press, 2014.

Warfa, Hamse, Ali Kofiro, Habon Abdulle, Zuhur Ahmed, Osman Ahmed, Abdirahman Ahmed, and Saida Hassan. "Somalis + Minnesota." *Minnesota History* 66, no. 1 (2018): 20–25.

WCCO CBS Minnesota. "Beverly Burrell to Receive No Additional Prison Time for 2 More Heroin Deaths." June 21, 2019. https://minnesota.cbslocal.com/2019/06/21/beverly-burrell-to-receive-no-additional-prison-time-for-two-heroin-deaths/.

WCCO-TV. "Hennepin Avenue, 1978." 1978. https://tcmedianow.com/wcco-tv-hennepin-avenue-1978/.

Weinmeyer Richard. "Needle Exchange Programs' Status in US Politics." *AMA Journal of Ethics* 18, no. 3 (2016): 252–57. https://doi.org/10.1001/journalofethics.2016.18.3.hlaw1-1603.

White, William. "Lessons of Language." In *Altering American Consciousness: The History of Alcohol and Drug Use in the United States, 1800–2000,* edited by Sarah W. Tracy and Caroline Jean Acker, 33–60. Amherst: University of Massachusetts Press, 2004.

———. "Narcotics Anonymous and the Pharmacotherapeutic Treatment of Opioid Addiction in the United States." Philadelphia Department of Behavioral Health and Intellectual disAbility Services and the Great Lakes Addiction Technology Transfer Center, 2011.

———. *Slaying the Dragon: The History of Addiction Treatment and Recovery in America*. 2nd ed. Bloomington, Ill.: Chestnut Health Systems Publication, 1998.

Wilhide, Anduin. "Somali and Somali American Experiences in Minnesota." MNopedia. Last modified December 5, 2018. https://www.mnopedia.org/somali-and-somali-american-experiences-minnesota.

Williams, Sarah T. "Legislative Path to Preventing Heroin Deaths Paved with Tears." *MinnPost*. April 23, 2014. https://www.minnpost.com/mental-health-addiction/2014/04/legislative-path-preventing-heroin-deaths-paved-tears/.

Wilson, Nana, Mbabazi Kariisa, Puja Seth, Herschel Smith IV, and Nicole L. Davis. "Drug and Opioid-Involved Overdose Deaths—United States, 2017–2018." *Morbidity and Mortality Weekly Report* 69 (2020): 290–97. http://dx.doi.org/10.15585/mmwr.mm6911a4.

Wood, Evan, Jeffrey H. Samet, and Nora D. Volkow. "Physician Education in Addiction Medicine." JAMA 310, no. 16 (2013): 1673–74.

Wren, Christopher S. "Clinton Calls Fashion Ads' 'Heroin Chic' Deplorable." *New York Times*. U.S. section. May 22, 1997. https://www.nytimes.com/1997/05/22/us/clinton-calls-fashion-ads-heroin-chic-deplorable.html.

Wysong, Earl, Richard Aniskiewicz, and David Wright. "Truth and DARE: Tracking Drug Education to Graduation and as Symbolic Politics." *Social Problems* 41, no. 3 (1994): 448–72. http://doi.org/10.2307/3096972.

Yussuf, Haji. "Goodbye, St. Cloud. I Love You, But I Can't Stand the Hate." *Sahan Journal*. August 11, 2019. https://sahanjournal.com/commentary/goodbye-st-cloud-i-love-you-but-i-cant-stand-the-hate/.

Yusuf, Ahmed Ismail. *Somalis in Minnesota*. The People of Minnesota. St. Paul: Minnesota Historical Society Press, 2012.

Zarefsky, Marc. "As COVID-19 Surges, AMA Sounds Alarm on Nation's Overdose Epidemic." American Medical Association. December 14, 2020. https://www.ama-assn.org/delivering-care/opioids/covid-19-surges-ama-sounds-alarm-nation-s-overdose-epidemic.

Index

Amy C. Sullivan, PhD, is an independent scholar and history professor at Macalester College in St. Paul, Minnesota. Her teaching and research focus on personal narratives, community healing, and social change via oral history, public history, and digital archive projects. She lives in Minneapolis with her family.